To my family and friends for their support and encouragement and especially to Ken,
who is always there to listen.
M.A.F.

To André, for his continued support.
G.K.C-G.

To Ron
J.J.B.

and *to all nurses, past, present, and future,*
who are dedicated to caring for the orthopaedic patient.
M.A.F.
G.K.C-G.
J.J.B.

Preface

In the current setting of health care delivery, which is becoming more technical, the basic concepts of care still exist. Traction has been used to manage a variety of orthopaedic conditions throughout the centuries, yet the fundamental principles of traction have not changed, although the appliances used have taken on a more modern appearance.

Now, the challenge of caring for a patient in traction is integrating the needed care into a more complex setting. The principles of care for the patient in traction are founded on basic holistic care principles. When concentrating on patient needs in relation to overall assessed needs, one must plan the care to incorporate all modalities being used.

This view holds true for both the patient in an intensive care unit and the patient at home. Each setting can be "complex," one because of the complexity of the environment and the other because of its simplicity. However, no matter where care is delivered, traction management is the same. It is the patient who is unique.

The book is intended to give readers a basic knowledge related to traction: the assessment of a patient in traction, the application of traction, basic principles related to the types of traction, and information needed to manage the patient in traction. It has been written to follow the nursing process.

The book addresses the care of patients in traction on a general unit as well as in a special-care area and in the home. Each type of traction is explained covering the following points:

1. A definition and brief description of the traction
2. An illustration of the traction, when applicable
3. The mechanical components of the specific traction:
   a. The angles of the system
   b. The weights
   c. The pulleys
   d. Countertraction
4. Nursing care specific to each type of traction including assessment, planning and interventions
5. Potential complications specific to the applied traction

Each chapter contains specific care guides to facilitate treatment of the patient in traction by allowing the practitioner to follow a systematic approach to reviewing the component parts of a traction apparatus as it is applied to the patient.

Who should read this book? Health care providers who assess and manage patients in traction will appreciate its value. Although its language is nursing oriented, physical therapists and others who may work with patients in traction will also find it invaluable.

A glossary of traction and orthopaedic terms will allow the novice and the expert to access terms and their specific meanings.

This book, focused on patient care and based on the nursing process, is intended to facilitate the care of patients in traction by giving health care professionals needed scientific knowledge in an easily readable format. We hope it has accomplished this purpose.

Marilyn A. Folcik, RN, MPH, ONC
Geraldine Carini-Garcia, RN
Jacqueline J. Birmingham, RN, MS, ACCC

Acknowledgments

With any major undertaking, there are many individuals who deserve recognition. The authors would like to acknowledge with sincere appreciation the assistance and support of the following people in the preparation of this book:

Dr. Robert L. Fisher, Former Chief of Orthopaedic Surgery, Hartford Hospital, Attending Orthopaedic Surgeon, Hartford Hospital, and Clinical Professor of Orthopaedic Surgery, University of Connecticut School of Medicine, for review of the manuscript.

André Garcia, whose drawings in the original text served as a basis for the present illustrations.

Jim Fox, Former Orthopaedic Technician, Hartford Hospital, for his help in setting up traction apparatus to be used for the illustrations.

Dr. Harry R. Gossling, Professor and Chairman Emeritus of the Department of Orthopaedic Surgery, University of Connecticut School of Medicine, Chairman of the Board of Directors, New Britain Memorial Hospital, New Britain, Connecticut, for review of the original text.

Marilyn A. Folcik, RN, MPH, ONC
Geraldine Carini-Garcia, RN
Jacqueline J. Birmingham, RN, MS, ACCC

Contents

Traction

ASSESSMENT AND MANAGEMENT

What Is Traction?

Traction is the application of a pulling force to a part of the body. The process can be used to treat injuries to the spine, long bones of the upper extremity, pelvis, and long bones of the lower extremity. Traction devices are applied externally, attached directly to bone and the skin.

Traction is used to treat
- Fractures (reduction and alignment)
- Contractures of muscles (deformities)
- Muscle spasms

Traction may also be used to
- Reduce a dislocated joint
- Immobilize a fracture and maintain alignment until callus formation and calcification begin
- Prevent further soft tissue damage
- Rest a diseased joint
- Hold a bone or bones in place for joint healing (e.g., traction for a fractured acetabulum)

Fractures

Traction is used both as a temporary measure before surgical intervention to repair a fracture and as a definitive treatment method. Traction can correct and maintain skeletal alignment so healing can occur. It also helps to immobilize the fracture, prevent further soft tissue damage at the fracture site, and reduce muscle spasm. As a result the pain associated with one or more fractures can be reduced.

When fractures of long bones occur, the muscles attached to the bones go into spasm and contract, possibly causing the bone fragments to become displaced (i.e., moved out of anatomical position). The sharp fragments of the broken bones can damage soft tissue, including the surrounding blood vessels, causing a hematoma (Fig. 1-1). Bone fragments may also damage nerves near the fracture site. The degree of displacement of the fracture ends depends on the mechanism of injury as well as the strength of the surrounding muscles. The displacement is described as sideways, angulated, overriding, rotated, or offset. Displacement results in deformity and shortening of the extremity. The application of traction helps to counteract muscle contraction and return the fracture fragments into anatomical position (Fig. 1-2).

Contractures and Spasms

Traction is used in the treatment of muscle contractures occurring as a result of poliomyelitis, muscular dystrophy, or other neuromuscular diseases. The pulling force of the traction stretches the shortened fibers of the contracted muscles or tendons over time and

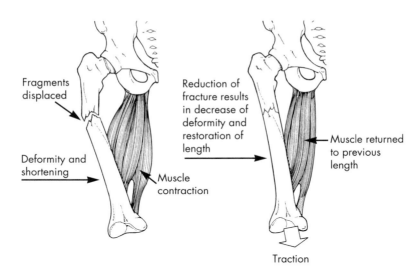

Figure 1-1   Application of traction to a long bone fracture.

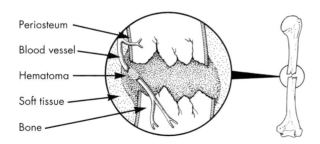

Figure 1-2   Fracture of a long bone.

thus helps to straighten the limb into a more functional position.

Traction is also used to treat muscle spasms. The pulling force of traction prevents muscles from developing spasmodic contractions or reduces the spasm, thereby decreasing pain as well.

Traction Mechanics

The mechanical components of traction include angles, weights, pulleys, and countertraction.

Angles. The physician determines the angles of the specific traction based on the type of injury. The placement of the pulleys on the bed frame and the angle of the involved joints determine the *line of pull*. This line must be along the *axis* of the bone, which is defined as the line that passes through the center of the body or a part of the body, such as the femoral axis (Fig. 2-1).

Weights. The physician prescribes the amount of weight that must be applied to provide the traction necessary to return the fracture fragments to as near anatomical position as possible. The weights are attached securely to a weight holder or are confined within a weight bag attached to a rope. The weights must hang freely and not be allowed to rest on the bed frame or the floor. The amount of weight applied determines the pulling force (traction). Too much weight can

1. Separate the bone fragments too far and thus prevent the fracture from healing. Bones heal faster if the ends of the fragments are in proximity. When the ends are too far away, no callus formation occurs.
2. Damage the surrounding soft tissue, blood vessels, and nerves. If the soft tissues stretch, the fibers sustain even more damage.
3. Increase pain. The soft tissue injury increases the amount of pain.

Too little weight can

1. Allow continued overriding of the bone fragments. This can result in shortening of the extremity and malunion (healing in a faulty position) of the fracture.
2. Allow motion at the fracture site. The right amount of weight stresses the surrounding muscle enough to keep the fragments in place and therefore allows for minimal motion at the fracture site.
3. Increase pain from muscle spasm. If the fragments are not held securely in place, their movement will allow muscles to contract, perhaps increasing soft tissue damage and therefore increasing the amount of pain.

Factors that influence the amount of weight to be applied include

- The fracture site. A fractured femur, surrounded by strong thigh muscles, will require more weight than a fractured humerus.
- The patient's age and weight. A femoral fracture in a 95-pound 15-year-old girl will require less weight than a femoral fracture in a 160-pound 20-year-old man.
- The strength of the muscle mass surrounding the fracture. A person who is athletic and

has well-developed quadriceps muscles will likely require more weight to reduce a fractured femur because the weight must counteract a greater muscle contraction than is found among the general population.

- The patient's medical condition. A person who has a bone disease or poor bone stock secondary to malnutrition or osteoporosis

will most likely be treated with less weight, especially if skeletal traction is used. Because the bone is soft, the pin could cut through the bone or the bone could fracture at the pin site.

Pulleys. The number of pulleys in the traction assembly affects the pull exerted. With one pulley, the traction force is equal to the amount of weight applied (Fig. 2-2). With two pulleys, the traction force exerted is twice the amount of weight applied (Fig. 2-3).

The number and position of the pulleys, which are securely fastened to the bed frame, are determined by the type of traction being used and are changed only upon order of the physician.

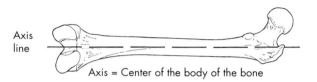

Figure 2-1   The axis of the bone determines the line of pull.

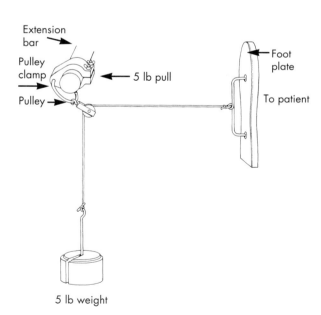

Figure 2-2   One pulley: traction force equals the amount of weight applied.

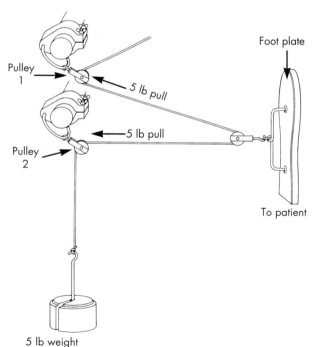

Figure 2-3   Two pulleys: traction force equals twice the amount of weight applied.

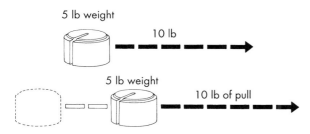

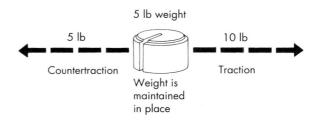

Figure 2-4   Countertraction in the same direction is a stable point from which the force of traction can pull.

Figure 2-5   Countertraction in the opposite direction.

Countertraction. Effective traction requires countertraction (i.e., a stable point from which the force of traction can pull). Countertraction can also be a pull in the direction opposite the pulling force of traction. If 10 pounds of pulling force is exerted on an object that weighs 5 pounds, the object will move toward the pulling force (Fig. 2-4). If 10 pounds of force is exerted on an object that weighs 5 pounds, but there is an added 5 pounds of pull in the opposite direction, the object will not move because equal forces will be opposing each other (Fig. 2-5). When a pulling force (traction) is applied to a part of the body, the weight of the body can act as a pulling force in the opposite direction (countertraction). To provide countertraction, the side or end of the bed toward the traction pull may be elevated. Countertraction may also be accomplished by using weights and ropes attached to a splint and then to the head of the bed (balanced- suspension traction).

3 General Nursing Management

Equipment

Maintaining effective traction includes maintaining the angles, weights, pulleys, and countertraction. This chapter explains the various components of traction and what you, the nurse, must know to maintain the traction properly. This chapter covers traction in a general sense. Specific care and maintenance will be covered in subsequent chapters that focus on each type of traction.

Equipment used when traction is applied includes a wide variety of items (Fig. 3-1).

Firm mattress. A firm mattress helps to maintain proper body alignment by providing adequate support for the body and preventing sagging of body parts.

Side rails. To provide safety for patients who are confused and/or disoriented, beds must have side rails. Side rails also provide security and support for patients who are allowed to turn, as in Buck's traction.

Bed frame and trapeze. A traction frame must be used to affix the traction to the bed. All orthopaedic beds should be equipped with an overhead frame, which is the base on which the traction is built. Several types of frames are available.

The patient uses the trapeze, which is attached to the overhead frame, to facilitate movement. The trapeze is routinely attached to all frames unless the patient's condition contradicts its use (e.g., cervical injuries are present).

Weights. Several methods are available for applying weight to maintain the traction pull and/or countertraction. Cast iron weights come in 1-, 2-, and 5-pound sizes and can be placed directly on weight holders or in specially made canvas bags. Sand bag weights come in 1-, 2-, 5-, and 10-pound sizes. The Zimmer Company manufacturers bags that can be filled with either sand or water and come in 5- and 10-pound capacities.

The weights must hang freely to maintain effective traction. Check frequently to ensure that weights have not become caught on part of the bed frame or are resting on the floor. As a safety precaution, weights should **never** hang over the patient. If the rope should fray and break, the patient could be injured.

Pulleys. A pulley is a small wheel with a grooved rim that is used with a rope to change the direction and point of application of a pulling force. Pulleys can be also used in combinations to increase the applied force. Pulleys allow the traction force to be maintained while the patient exercises some degree of mobility.

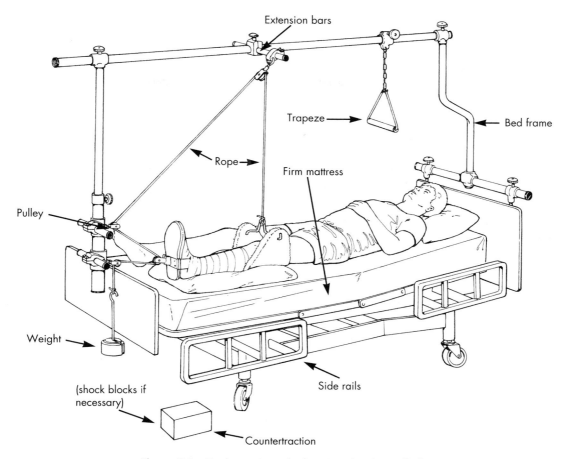

Figure 3-1 Equipment used when traction is applied.

The pulleys must be securely attached to the bed frame in the appropriate positions, which are determined by the physician and the type of injury. Check the wheel of the pulley frequently to make sure it moves freely, thus helping to promote effective traction.

Rope. Traction rope or cord is made of braided polyester or nylon fibers. The rope or cord must be in the groove of the wheel of the pulley. Check it frequently for fraying, kinking, and stretching. To prevent slipping, tape all knots in the rope or cord that are tied to either a frame or a weight holder. When the traction is discontinued, discard the rope or cord; it should not be reused. This helps to ensure that it will be strong enough to sustain the amount of weight for effective traction.

Countertraction. Countertraction is essential to maintain effective traction. It can be accomplished using the patient or part of the patient's body, positioning the bed, or using weights pulling in the opposite direction. If the pulling force of the traction is greater than the amount of countertraction, the patient will slide toward the traction force, which can cause impingement of the traction apparatus on the pulley and subsequently negate the traction pull. More countertraction may be needed and can be supplied by keeping the patient in good body alignment and not allowing the head of the bed to be elevated more than 20 to 30 degrees. Another method of increasing countertraction is to tilt the bed away from the traction force. This can be accomplished by elevating the foot of the bed electrically into Trendelenburg position or by placing blocks under the wheels of the bed, depending on the type of bed available.

Applying Traction

Traction is usually applied by the physician or a trained orthopaedic technician. Depending on the institution, you may be responsible for applying Buck's traction. However, you must know which application technique will facilitate care of the patient. This section is an overview of the basic traction modalities. In-depth discussion of the various types of traction will be offered in subsequent chapters.

The pulling force of traction can be applied to the body manually or mechanically. Both methods are discussed here.

Manual Traction

In manual traction the pulling force is applied directly to the extremity by hand contact; hence the term "manual." The physician exerts a strong steady pull on the extremity to return the fractured bone to an anatomical position. This is a temporary type of traction and is used mainly as a preliminary mechanism before traction or a cast is applied. This type of traction is also used to reduce dislocated joints (Fig. 3-2).

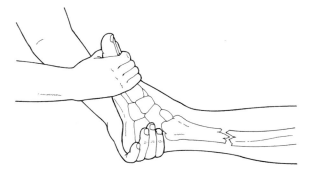

Figure 3-2   Application of manual traction.

Mechanical Traction

Mechanical traction, meaning that which is mechanically attached to the patient, includes both skin and skeletal traction. The method of applying the traction depends on factors such as the following: (1) the type and location of the injury (e.g., cervical vs femoral fractures), (2) any associated injuries (open or compound fractures vs closed or simple fractures), and (3) the physician's preference (halo traction vs cervical tongs).

Skin traction. In skin traction a pulling force is applied directly to the patient's skin and soft tissues, immobilizing the body part. Skin traction is used in the treatment of fractures that require a minimal amount of traction pull over a relatively short period. Skin traction may be intermittent and can be used in the treatment of fractures before surgical intervention or the application of skeletal traction.

Skin traction can be applied using adhesive traction straps that are wrapped with elastic bandages. If this form is used, the traction is usually not to be removed unless a problem arises (e.g., skin breakdown or traction slippage). Another method of applying skin traction is to use commercially available foam rubber traction boots, belts, or halters. These can be more easily removed and replaced with minimal effect on the skin. Whichever modality is used, strict adherence to the institution's standard of care for maintenance of skin integrity is essential. Appropriate nursing interventions must be incorporated into the daily nursing care.

Chapter 4 offers a more in-depth discussion of the types of skin traction and the associated nursing care.

Skeletal traction. In skeletal traction the pulling force is applied directly to the bone by pins, wires, screws, or tongs. Skeletal traction is very efficient because the pulling force is exerted directly on the bones involved and does not have to be transferred through the skin or soft tissues. Skeletal traction allows the use of larger amounts of weight over a longer period. This type of traction not only facilitates reduction of the fracture but also can control for rotation of the fracture fragments.

Skeletal traction is used when

1. A large muscle mass surrounds the fracture (e.g., a fractured femur). The ability to use more weight helps to counteract the strong contractions of the large thigh muscles.
2. The weight required to maintain reduction of a fracture is greater than what can safely be applied to the skin. The maximum amount of weight for skin traction on arms and legs is 5 to 8 pounds for adults and 1 to 5 pounds for children. When more weight is applied, the risks of small blood vessel occlusion and skin breakdown increase. Skeletal traction can accommodate 15 to 40 pounds of weight depending on the type of injury, body part affected, body size, and type of bone stock.
3. Fractures of long bones cannot be immediately repaired surgically (e.g., a fractured femur in a patient who is medically unstable secondary to other injuries, such as a closed head injury or chest injury).
4. Rotation of the fracture must be controlled. This can be accomplished by adjusting the weights and pulleys directly on the pin or wire to tilt or twist the fragments into a more anatomical position.
5. An open or compound fracture of a long bone exists. In this case the wound may be contaminated. The introduction and placement of hardware to fix the fracture internally would be contraindicated because of the increased risk of infection and osteomyelitis.
6. An unstable fracture of a long bone has fragments that can be displaced in a cast. By applying skeletal traction, the fragments can be maintained in alignment until healing starts and callus formation is evident on roentgenograms (x-rays). At this time, cast application is considered to allow the patient more mobility.
7. An unstable dislocation must be held in place until healing occurs or surgical intervention is safe (e.g., dislocation of a cervical vertebra or fracture-dislocation of the acetabulum).

Equipment for skeletal traction. As with determining the amount of weight, determining the equipment to be used for skeletal traction varies depending on the type of injury, body part affected, patient's size, and type of bone stock.

1. Pins and wires. The most commonly used pins and wires are the Steinmann pin and the

Kirschner wire. Each is used for a specific type of skeletal traction. (Fig. 3-3).

The Steinmann pin has a relatively large diameter. It is used in the treatment of fractures of the femur because it is strong enough to withstand considerable weight without bending. These pins are usually made of stainless steel and are inserted using sterile technique with the patient under anesthesia.

The Kirschner wire is smaller in diameter than the Steinmann pin and, because of this, is not used with heavy weights. One advantage of the Kirschner wire is that because of its smaller diameter, insertion requires a smaller opening in the skin, resulting in destruction of fewer bone cells and also decreasing the risk of pin track infection. These wires are also made out of stainless steel and are inserted using sterile technique and local anesthesia.

2. Halo and tongs. Halo and tongs are used specifically in the treatment of cervical fractures and dislocations, in the treatment of cervical spondylosis, or before an anterior interbody fusion to increase the intervertebral space. Other devices are also available.

The halo and tongs are directly embedded into the skull using stainless steel pins. Tongs are attached to weights of up to 35 pounds. Bedrest is required for the patient being treated with cervical tong traction. Caution must be used when turning the patient and providing care to maintain the traction and alignment and to prevent further injury to the patient.

The cervical halo is applied in the same manner as the cervical tongs; however, a jacket of either plaster or polyurethane plastic may be attached to the halo with four bars extending from the jacket to the halo. This apparatus allows the patient to be mobile while maintain-

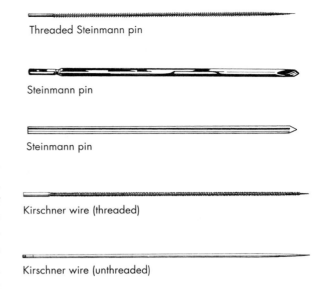

Threaded Steinmann pin

Steinmann pin

Steinmann pin

Kirschner wire (threaded)

Kirschner wire (unthreaded)

Figure 3-3   Pins and wires commonly used in skeletal traction.

ing stability of the cervical vertebrae. A more detailed discussion is provided in Chapter 7.

When skeletal traction is applied, it is maintained until healing occurs, the fracture is surgically repaired, or the physician discontinues the treatment. If the traction is interrupted, severe muscle spasm may result and cause loss of alignment of the fracture fragments. This could increase the patient's pain and possibly further injure the soft tissues, blood vessels, and nerves. Further discussion of skeletal traction can be found in Chapter 6.

3. External fixator. Another method of fracture management is the Hoffman or Ilizarov apparatus. Although not complying with all principles of traction, the fixators are used for reduction of fractures and embody the principles of distraction as well as compression and immobilization.

An external fixator consists of several wires or pins placed into or through the bone above and below the fracture site. An external device or outrigger is then attached to the pins or wires to stabilize the fracture and maintain immobilization. This method of treatment allows for early ambulation and therefore decreases the risks associated with immobilization. Further discussion of external fixators can be found in Chapter 8.

.... ▼ ....

C A R E   G U I D E

GENERAL TRACTION MANAGEMENT

MECHANICAL COMPONENTS

1. Weights . . . .
   - a. Prescribed amount by doctor
   - b. Secure
   - c. Hanging freely
     - (1) Not caught on bed
     - (2) Not caught on frame
     - (3) Not on floor
     - (4) Not hanging over patient
   - d. At least 12 inches from pulley

2. Pulleys . . . .
   - a. Securely attached to bed frame
   - b. Wheels move freely

3. Ropes . . . .
   - a. In groove of pulley
   - b. Freely movable
   - c. No fraying
   - d. No kinks
   - e. No unnecessary knots
   - f. Knots taped to prevent slipping

4. Countertraction . . . .
   - a. Countertraction provided by one of these methods
     - (1) 6-inch shock blocks
     - (2) Trendelenburg position
     - (3) Patient's body weight
     - (4) Sling support (Boehler-Braun)

5. Angles . . . .
   - a. Pulling force exerted along axis of bone
   - b. No adjustment made in location of pulleys or position of patient unless ordered by physician

6. Bed . . . .
   - a. Firm mattress
   - b. Siderails

         c. Bed boards (if necessary)
         d. Frame securely attached
         e. If therapeutic bed
            (1) Check cables
            (2) Check pads
            (3) Check surroundings for bed mobility, movement, etc.

7. Trapeze. . . . .
         a. Securely fastened to frame
         b. Hangs so patient's elbows are flexed 20 degrees when grasping trapeze
         c. Attached slightly anterior to level of patient's shoulders

PATIENT ALIGNMENT

1. Traction pull . . . .
         a. Traction apparatus is freely movable, not resting against pulley or bed frame
         b. Patient straight in bed
         c. All necessary items within reach of patient

2. Provision of comfort when moving patient
         a. Explain procedure to patient
         b. Teach patient how to use trapeze
         c. Use firm steady motion avoiding bumping or jarring of bed or traction apparatus
         d. Get help when necessary

MAINTENANCE OF SKIN INTEGRITY

1. Check pressure points . . . .
         a. General: sacrum, heels, coccyx, trochanters, spine, scapulae
         b. Upper extremity: epicondyles, olecrenon, ulna
         c. Lower extremity: Achilles tendon, malleoli, dorsum of foot, popliteal space, head of fibula
         d. Cervical: chin, back of head, ears, temporomandibular joint

2. Check for increased risk of skin breakdown
         a. Patients who are
            (1) Debilitated
            (2) Confused
            (3) Obese

    (4) Emaciated
    (5) Diabetic
    (6) Paralyzed
    (7) Incontinent
  b. Patients who have history of circulatory problems
  c. Patients who will be immobilized for prolonged period

3. Adjunct equipment to decrease risk of skin breakdown . . . .
  a. Special mattresses
    (1) Egg crate
    (2) Water
    (3) Air
    (4) Other
  b. Protectors for heels and elbows
  c. Pillow supports
  d. Sheepskin
  e. Therapeutic bed
  f. No "donut"-type devices

EVALUATION OF AFFECTED EXTREMITY

1. Alteration in tissue perfusion (circulation)
  a. Check pulses distal to injury or traction site
  b. Check capillary filling (normal 2 to 4 seconds)
  c. Observe for
    (1) Warmth
    (2) Color
    (3) Swelling
  d. Compare to opposite extremity
  e. Check for Homan's sign

2. Alteration in neurological status . . . .
  a. Check for motion of extremity and ability to dorsiflex foot
  b. Check for sensation:
    (1) Pressure and touch
    (2) Pain
    (3) Numbness
    (4) Tingling

NURSING CARE

1. Alteration in gas exchange . . . .
   a. Patient coughs and deep breathes
   b. Patient uses incentive spirometry correctly
   c. Suction and oxygen apparatus available if necessary

2. Alteration in nutritional status . . . .
   a. Patient eats well-balanced diet
   b. Patient drinks adequate fluids
   c. Provide supplements as necessary

3. Alteration in elimination . . . .
   a. Encourage fluids
   b. Check for urinary retention
      (1) Palpate bladder
      (2) Catheterize if necessary
   c. Establish pattern for elimination
      (1) Retraining program if needed
      (2) Offer bed pan on regular schedule
      (3) Provide privacy
      (4) Use fracture pan
      (5) Record intake and output

4. Ineffective coping . . . .
   a. Explain all procedures
   b. Allow patient to verbalize
   c. Encourage involvement of family and friends
   d. Provide diversional activities
   e. Investigate for home or family difficulty that might require intervention (discharge planning)
   f. Access resources as necessary

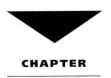

4 Skin Traction to the Lower Extremity and Hip

Skin traction involves applying a pulling force to the skin and soft tissue of the injured or diseased part of the body. The pull is created by using strips of moleskin or adhesive applied directly to the skin or by using commercial skin traction strips (Fig. 4-1). Commercial boots (Buck's and Russell's traction) (Fig. 4-2) or belts (pelvic traction) may also be used. The benefit of using a boot or belt is that it can be removed and replaced periodically to facilitate skin care whereas strips adhere directly to the skin and repeated removal or slippage can cause irritation and possible breakdown of the tissues.

The major indication for skin traction in adult patients is the treatment of fractures or dislocations that do not require a large amount of weight or a long period of immobilization. In children, skin traction may be used to treat certain fractures and dislocations because it is better tolerated than skeletal traction.

Buck's Extension Traction

Buck's extension is an example of straight line traction (Fig. 4-3). Traction is applied to the extremity and attached to weights through a pulley, creating a pull in only one direction—a straight line from the affected extremity. When Buck's extension is applied, 1 pound of weight equals 1 pound of force (traction). If 5 pounds of weight is applied, 5 pounds of pull is placed on the extremity (Fig. 4-4).

Buck's extension traction applies a pulling force to the skin of the lower extremity and is

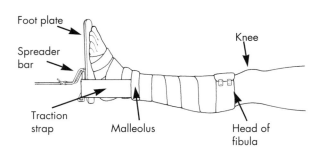

Figure 4-1 Moleskin adhesive skin traction strips.

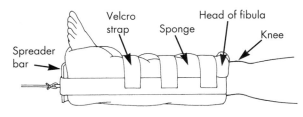

Figure 4-2 Commercial boot.

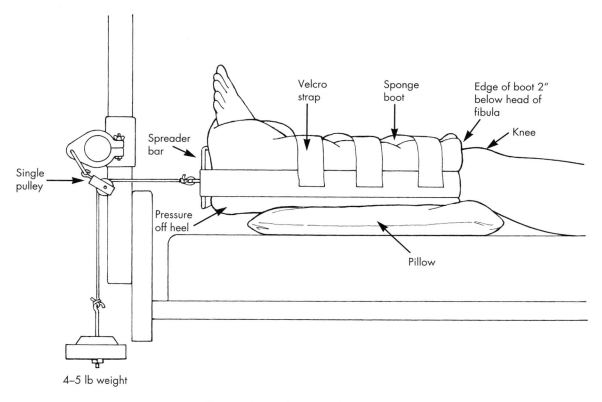

Figure 4-3   Buck's extension traction.

often used in the temporary treatment of fractures. It may be used for immobilization and pain control while the patient is being evaluated for surgery. The amount of weight chosen for this type of traction in an adult is usually 5 pounds and should not exceed 8 pounds, because the skin will not tolerate it. Limiting the weight decreases the risk of skin abrasions or other breakdown. Buck's extension is not used for reduction of fractures or if traction is to be maintained for more than 3 to 4 weeks. If limb rotation is a primary concern in the treatment of the fracture, a different method of traction should be considered.

Mechanical Components

Angles: The pulling force is applied with the leg in a straight line. A pillow* under the leg is used to keep pressure off the heel.

---

*The placement of a **flat** pillow or bath blanket under the affected extremity is a controversial point. It does not appear to alter the straight line of pull significantly. However, it does allow the heel of the affected extremity to clear the bed, relieving pressure on the heel and therefore reducing the risk of skin breakdown. We suggest that when applying Buck's traction or caring for a patient in Buck's traction you clarify the placement of a pillow or bath blanket with hospital policy and/or physician preference. We also recommend using a pillow as seen in Figure 4-3.

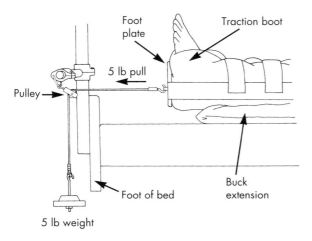

Figure 4-4   Buck's traction (5 lb weight = 5 lb pull).

Weight. As already stated, the weight is usually 5 pounds and should not exceed 8 pounds.

Pulleys. Buck's extension uses a single pulley system (i.e., one pulley attached to the frame at the end of the bed).

Countertraction. Countertraction is provided by elevating the foot of the bed approximately 6 inches or by using the patient's own body weight.

Russell's Traction

Russell's traction is also used for the lower extremity, but two pulling forces are applied to the fractured extremity. One force is applied by a double-pulley system at the foot. The other is applied in an upward direction using a sling under the knee attached by a rope to a single overhead pulley (Fig. 4-5). The result of these two forces pulling in different directions is a pull in a third direction (vectors of force principle). (See Figure 4-5.)

Russell's traction is based on the principles of a parallelogram. The pulling force in line with the lower leg (Fig. 4-6), *A–D*, and the upward pull from the knee, *A–B*, create a force along the axis of the femur, *A–C*. The line of pull is also referred to as the **vector of force**. Russell's traction supports the leg in a position that allows continuous pull in line with the femur. By keeping the knee flexed, and supporting the leg on a pillow, the traction can control angulation and rotatory deformity of the fracture. Russell's traction is not recommended for treatment of fractures of the shaft of the femur because it provides no protection for bone fragments against backward sagging or lateral angulation.

Mechanical Components

Angles. The physician arranges the angles of the traction so the resultant pulling force is along the axis of the femur. The placement of the overhead pulley supporting the sling controls the direction of the pulling force. The angle between the thigh and the mattress should be maintained at approximately 20 degrees. This can be accomplished by placing a pillow under the affected extremity, making sure that the lower leg remains parallel to the bed.

Weight. The weight applied is usually 4 pounds for adults and ½ to 2 pounds for infants through older children. Effective traction is sometimes less than the applied weight because of friction from the pulleys and rope.

Pulleys. The two-pulley system at the foot doubles the amount of traction force applied to the leg (vectors of force principle). The overhead single pulley allows for adjustment of the sling to maintain the angle of the thigh to the bed at 20 degrees and to help maintain the resultant force on the axis of the femur.

Countertraction. Countertraction may be provided by the patient's own body weight or

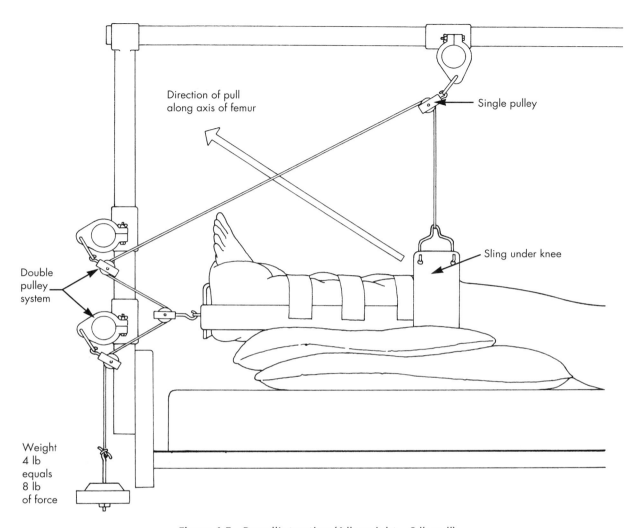

Figure 4-5   Russell's traction (4 lb weight = 8 lb pull).

by elevating the foot of the bed approximately 6 inches.

Bryant's Traction

Bryant's traction is specifically used in pediatric settings. It will be discussed separately at the end of this chapter.

Applying the Traction

Before Buck's or Russell's traction is applied, the patient's skin should be assessed. Because traction involves mechanical apparatus that may incorporate factors like shearing forces, pressure, and restraint, the patient's skin is at risk of breaking down. If the patient is physi-

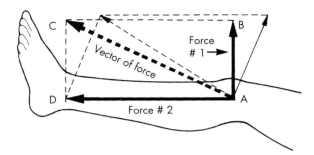

Figure 4-6 Vector of force: the pulling forces along lines *A-B* and *A-D* create the force of *A-C* along the axis of the femur.

cally immobilized, elderly, and medically compromised, this risk increases.

In most institutions the physician or specifically trained personnel must apply all forms of traction used for the reduction and maintenance of fracture alignment. However, a nurse may be required to apply Buck's traction for pain relief and reduction of muscle spasms. Certain factors must be considered before applying any type of skin traction:

- Do not apply it over an open wound or on an abraded, lacerated, blistered, or infected extremity.
- Ask the patient or family about any allergies to adhesive (if traction strips are used) or to rubber (if the foam rubber boot is applied).
- Use traction adhesive strips only after careful consideration of the patient's neurovascular status and skin integrity.

If adhesive strips are used (Fig. 4-2), remember the following points:

1. Shaving the extremity may be needed before application, especially if the patient is male.
2. When applying the traction strips, make sure the sticky side contacts the skin

above the malleoli and ends below the head of the fibula. Because these areas are bony prominences and at risk of skin breakdown, pad them well using soft bandages (e.g., Webril).

3. Once the strips are in place, wrap an elastic bandage around the leg to secure them. When wrapping the bandage, be sure to include the foot and continue wrapping to the area just below the knee.
4. To be applied properly, the elastic bandage must start at the dorsum of the foot and continue around the leg with an even tension.
5. Make sure the footpiece of the pulley mechanism is wide enough so the strips do not cause pressure on the side of the foot.
6. Assess all bony prominences as well as all skin coming in contact with the strips.
7. Avoid pressure over the Achilles tendon, the malleoli, and the head of the fibula.
8. Give special attention to **both** heels.

If a commercial traction boot is used (Fig. 4-7), make sure that it is the correct size.

1. Estimate the patient's size and weight or ask the patient to estimate them.
2. Using a tape measure, measure the circumference of the widest part of the calf, approximately 2 inches below the knee joint line.
3. Sizes vary with manufacturers; however, the following may be helpful:
   Order a **small** size if the maximum calf circumference is less than 11.5 inches, a **medium** if it is between 11.5 and 13 inches, and a **large** if it is between 13 and 14.5 inches.

Most commercial boots are one length (approximately 17 inches). When applying the

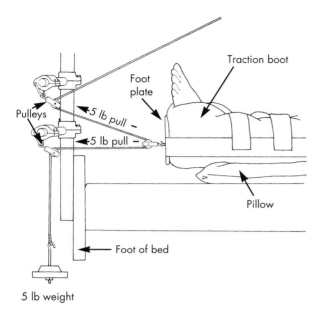

Figure 4-7 Commercial traction boot.

boot, make sure that the top of the boot does **not** cover the back of the knee. This helps to decrease the risk of vascular problems.

To apply the boot, follow this procedure:

1. Place the bare leg on a flat pillow.
2. After thoroughly assessing the extremity, gently lift the leg slightly to slide the open boot into place.
3. Fold the sides over each other and then fasten the Velcro straps snugly but not overly tight.
4. When applying the traction, make sure that the footpiece is correctly in place (Fig. 4-7) and that it is securely fastened.
5. Tie the traction rope to the footpiece, threading the loose end through the pulley placed on the crossbar of the frame at the end of the bed.
6. Tie the rope to the weight bag or weight holder.

7. Gently apply the prescribed amount of weight, being careful not to drop the weight or jar the patient.

Open the traction boot periodically to examine the skin, give care, and evaluate the extremity for circulatory and neurological status. In addition, the heel may be repositioned in the boot. To reposition the heel:

1. Release the weights by lifting them gently and placing them on the bed or hanging them securely on the crossbar to maintain release.
2. Open the boot by unfastening the Velcro straps.
3. **Do not lift the leg out of the boot.**
4. Depress the sponge boot into the pillow so you can see the area clearly to inspect the heel and provide care
5. Do not put elastic stockings on the affected leg.

RELATED NURSING DIAGNOSES

Impaired Physical Mobility: Related to prolonged bedrest

Assessment	Rationale
Assess alignment of affected extremity	Patient should be straight in bed with extremity in neutral position to avoid discomfort
Assess alignment of entire body	Maintains optimum efficiency of traction
Assess tightness of elastic bandages or traction boot	Decreases risk of neurovascular impairment
Assess skin	Any foul odor or drainage from traction site may indicate skin breakdown

Assessment

Assess neurovascular status:
    Circulation
    Motion
    Sensation

Assess for signs and symptoms of deep venous thrombosis (DVT)

Assess respiratory status

Assess proper method of ambulation (e.g., weight-bearing vs non-weight-bearing, walker vs crutches vs cane)

Rationale

Provides for timely intervention if impairment is noted

Provides for timely interventions

May indicate pulmonary problems

Beginning ambulation as soon as possible will help to reduce risk of complications resulting from immobilization

Interventions

1. Protect the affected extremity while promoting and maintaining the function of other joints.

2. Devise an exercise program taking into consideration the injury and type of traction being used.

3. Teach the patient to participate in passive and active exercises as able.

4. Encourage the patient to perform as many activities of daily living (ADLs) as possible. This promotes motion, increases the patient's self-esteem, and allows the patient to exert some control over the situation.

5. If the patient can exercise alone, include active-assistive exercises to the unaffected extremity on a regular basis. Lower extremity exercises that the patient may perform in bed include:

   a. **Dorsiflexion:** The patient flexes the ankle so the toes are directed toward the knee.

   b. **Plantarflexion:** The patient extends the ankle by pointing the toes downward.

   c. **Quadriceps setting ("quad setting"):** The patient tightens the muscles of the thigh by pushing the knee into the bed and

tightening the kneecap and thigh muscles. This is maintained for a count of 10 and then released.

   d. **Ankle circling:** The patient moves the ankle in a circular motion. This can be done with the leg lifted or flat on the bed.

   e. **Straight leg raising and knee bending:** The patient raises the unaffected leg without bending the knee and then bends the knee by pulling the heel toward the buttocks.

   f. **Range of motion:** Range of motion exercises to the upper extremities include flexion, extension, abduction, adduction, and circumduction of the hands, wrists, elbows, and shoulders. The best exercise for the upper extremity is patient participation in eating, bathing, and moving as much as possible. These activities also foster independence.

6. Auscultate the lungs at least every shift while the patient is confined to bed.

7. Encourage the patient to cough and deep-breathe and to use the incentive spirometer at least every 2 hours while awake.

8. Apply an elastic stocking to the unaffected extremity in an effort to decrease the risk of thrombophlebitis. Remove and reapply the stocking at least once per shift to assess the skin.

9. If the patient is being treated in Buck's traction, you may be able to turn him or her for skin inspection as well as positioning.

   a. Plan a schedule of turning every 2 hours while the patient is immobilized.

   b. At this time, thoroughly examine the coccygeal area and scapular regions.

   c. Although controversial, turning a patient in Buck's extension traction to the affected side can be accomplished without making the patient too uncomfortable.

   d. Turning the patient to the affected side

splints the fractured extremity against the bed and can bring the patient welcome relief.

To turn a patient in skin traction, follow these directions. **Note:** This procedure may require a physician's order. It also may be necessary to have more than one person available to complete the procedure.

1. Place the head of the bed in the flat position unless contraindicated.
2. Carefully remove the flat pillow or bath blanket from under the affected leg and place it between the patient's legs.
3. Supporting the patient's leg with the pillow, have the patient roll to one side like a log. Use of the trapeze or side rail for support is beneficial. Turning to the affected side is usually more comfortable for the patient.
4. While the patient is positioned in this manner, place pillows at the back and between the legs to enable the patient to remain for a short time.
5. Remember: When turning a patient in traction, move slowly. **Avoid quick and jerky movements.** This decreases the risk of pain and muscle spasms.

Alteration in Skin Integrity: Related to immobility

Assessment	Rationale
Assess skin integrity on admission to hospital	May need to change treatment plan if open areas are present or if skin integrity is compromised
Assess patient's complaints of discomfort	May indicate area of concern not evident on initial examination (e.g., a deep bruise)

Assessment	Rationale
Assess for swelling of extremity	Sites of constrictive bandages must be monitored to prevent development of compartment syndrome
Assess nutritional status and hydration	Patients who are malnourished or dehydrated are at increased risk of skin breakdown secondary to depleted protein stores and fluid deficiency
Assess mental status	Patients who are confused or agitated may be more prone to skin breakdown because of excessive movement; may also be prone to incontinence and noncompliance
Assess neurovascular status	May need to change treatment plan if neurovascular impairment is recognized

Interventions

1. Keep the skin dry and clean.
2. Inspect the skin for redness, cyanosis, blistering, temperature, and circulation at least every 2 hours initially.
3. Avoid pressure on bony prominences and other areas.
4. Turn and reposition the patient every 2 hours if tolerated.
5. Instruct the patient to lift the buttocks off the bed at least every 2 hours to change position and to relieve the pressure on the coccyx and buttocks. This can be accomplished by instructing the patient to bend the unaffected leg, place the foot flat on the mattress, and push down while lifting the buttocks off the bed. The patient may also use the trapeze.

6. Massage the coccyx and scapulae with a lubricant to keep the skin supple.

7. Massage the heels and other areas of the lower extremities. Pressure points that are especially vulnerable when the boot is being used are the dorsum of the foot, the heel, and the head of the fibula.

8. **Never** massage the calf of the leg, especially if it is painful and swollen, because if a DVT (deep vein thrombosis) exists the possibility of dislodging it increases.

9. Avoid excessive pressure on the skin by using special mattresses, sheepskins, positioning of the patient with pillows, special protectors (for heel and elbow), or a therapeutic bed.

10. Avoid using "donuts" or rubber rings. These appliances tend to restrict the circulation to the coccyx, which increases the risk of skin breakdown.

11. Decrease shearing forces on the coccyx by not elevating the head of the bed more than 30 degrees.

12. Encourage the patient to eat a diet that provides adequate amounts of protein and calories.

13. Encourage adequate fluid intake to prevent dehydration. Suggested total intake is approximately 2600 ml per 24 hours for a patient without medical restrictions.

14. Reinforce orientation as to time, place, and self if needed.

15. Have family members bring in familiar objects and pictures.

16. Keep a small light on to maintain orientation at night.

Pain: Related to fracture

Assessment	Rationale
Assess for signs and symptoms of pain or discomfort related to site and severity	May indicate that treatment is not appropriate or that traction is improperly applied

Assessment	Rationale
	Indicates need to offer or administer analgesics
	May indicate possible complications (e.g., DVT or thrombophlebitis)

Interventions

1. Administer analgesics as ordered, making sure to document the patient's response.

2. Teach the patient to use alternative methods of pain control to augment the use of analgesics, including relaxation techniques and diversional activities such as reading, watching TV, or listening to the radio.

3. Reposition, turn, or readjust the traction as necessary to decrease discomfort.

Self-Care Deficits: Related to immobility and pain

Assessment	Rationale
Assess for ability to perform activities of daily living (ADLs)	Needed for determining level of activity (i.e., Does patient need to be fed? Can patient bathe? Can patient use urinal or bedpan?)

Interventions

1. Assist the patient with self-care activities as needed.

2. Position the patient for these activities, keeping necessary equipment within reach and avoiding awkward or uncomfortable positions.

3. Place the overbed stand within reach and the bedside stand on the unaffected side. This allows the patient to reach necessary equipment, increasing independence and perhaps self-esteem.

4. Encourage the patient to perform as many functions as possible.

Altered Patterns of Elimination (Incontinence or Retention and Constipation): Related to immobilization and altered nutritional status

Assessment	Rationale
Assess for incontinence, retention, or constipation	Incontinence can lead to skin breakdown and constipation can cause impaction, so normal elimination pattern should be established as soon as possible
Assess intake and output	May indicate need for change in diet to promote normal bladder and bowel function

Interventions

1. Learn the patient's previous elimination habits.

2. Develop and implement a schedule to train the bladder while the patient is on bedrest.

3. Provide privacy.

4. Keep the patient dry and clean to prevent skin breakdown.

5. Encourage the patient to maintain an adequate fluid intake to decrease the risk of renal calculi.

The following approach to offering the patient a bedpan is recommended:

1. Obtain a small "fracture pan."

2. If possible, have the patient help to lift by using the trapeze attached to the overhead frame.

3. Instruct the patient to bend the unaffected leg, put the foot flat on the mattress, and push down while lifting with the trapeze. This will raise the buttocks slightly.

4. While standing at the patient's unaffected side, place your hand under the patient's buttocks to make sure he lifts high enough to avoid scraping the coccyx on the bedpan.

5. Gently slide the bedpan under the patient.

6. Remove the pan using the same technique, after ensuring that the patient is clean and dry.

7. Make sure that the bed is clean and dry and that the bed sheet is unwrinkled.

Alternate method: If the patient is able to turn (e.g., in Buck extension traction), an alternate method may be used. NOTE: This method may require more than one person.

1. Remove the flat pillow or bath blanket from under the affected leg.

2. Place the pillow between the legs.

3. Supporting the affected leg, have the patient roll to one side using the side rail as a support. Usually moving to the affected side is more comfortable.

4. Position the pan under the buttocks.

5. Have the patient roll back onto the pan.

6. Remove the pan using the same technique.

7. Make sure that the patient and the bed are clean and dry and that the sheet is unwrinkled.

Impaired Gas Exchange: Related to bedrest

Assessment	Rationale
Assess respiratory status: auscultate lungs	Decreased breath sounds, rales or rhonchi, and wheezing may indicate hypostatic pneumonia
Assess vital signs, including temperature, respiration rate, dyspnea, congestion, and cyanosis	To allow early recognition of signs and symptoms of hypostatic pneumonia

Interventions

1. Use caution in administering drugs that may decrease the rate and depth of lung expansion and that suppress the cough reflex.

2. Observe the patient for signs and symptoms associated with hypostatic pneumonia: shortness of breath, elevated temperature, dyspnea, cyanosis, congestion, and lethargy.

3. Instruct and monitor the patient in using respiratory aid procedures such as incentive spirometry, coughing, and deep breathing. These help the patient to inhale deeply.

4. Do not allow the patient to smoke.

Ineffective Coping: Related to bedrest and hospitalization

Assessment	Rationale
Assess patient's ability to perform self-care activities; also note any change in emotional response	Disinterest in personal hygiene may indicate depression
Evaluate patient's support systems	Support from family and friends is important in self-esteem and motivating patient to get well

Interventions

1. Develop a rapport with the patient.

2. Be aware of the normal grieving responses and allow the patient to express feelings openly.

3. Be aware of the resources available to the patient and be able to access them in a timely fashion.

High Risk for Peripheral Vascular Impairment: Related to traction application and immobility

To assess for adequate circulatory status, do the following:

- Check the presence and quality of pulses distal to (below) the injury or traction application site.

- To check capillary filling, use the blanching sign, which evaluates arterial return. Gently pinch the skin or nail bed of the affected extremity below the injury or site of traction application. The nail bed or skin should "blanch," or turn white. However, as soon as the pressure of the pinch is eliminated, the area should return to its normal pink color. The presence or absence of capillary refill is indicated by how rapidly this occurs. If the skin does not return to its normal color within 2 to 4 seconds, suspect damage to the arterial circulation. Report and document these findings immediately. Poor capillary filling may indicate that the traction apparatus is applied too tightly or incorrectly or that there is an occult injury to the vascular system.

- Observe for swelling, warmth, and color. Some residual swelling from the original injury may exist, but the extremity should be warm to the touch and the color should be about the same as that of the unaffected extremity. If the extremity is cold to the touch, has a whitish blue appearance, or has whitish blue nail beds, vascular integrity may be compromised. Report and document these findings immediately.

- Ascertain if motion greatly increases pain. To do this, gently move the toes of the affected extremity. If the patient complains of extreme pain, beyond what is normal or expected, suspect compartment syndrome, a potentially limb-threatening condition resulting from compression of the nerves and vessels in the compartment of the extremity. This syndrome is explained in greater detail in Chapter 9.

To assess neurological status

- Ascertain if the patient is experiencing pain, numbness, tingling, or loss of sensation in the extremity. Check for any loss of sensation by lightly touching the extremity with your hand or an open paperclip, being careful not to break the skin. Causing a break in the skin would increase the risk of infection.
- Check for continued motor function. Ask the patient to move the toes of both feet.
- Ascertain if the patient can feel gentle pressure exerted on a point distal to (below) the injury or site of traction application.
- Document your findings and notify the physician immediately of any deficit in these areas.

Bryant's (Divarication) Traction for Pediatric Patients

Bryant's traction is the application of skin traction to both lower extremities (Fig. 4-8). It is used in children who are under the age of 3 years and weigh less than 35 pounds (17.5 kilograms). It is used primarily to treat patients with developmental dysplasia of the hip (DDH), formerly known as congenital dislocation of the hip (CDH). In DDH the head of the femur does not articulate in the center of the acetabulum and may be completely out of the socket. Bryant traction gradually reduces the dislocation, stretching the muscles and tendons and positioning the femoral head so it can be reduced. This use of Bryant traction is sometimes referred to as **divarication traction.** The term "divarication" means to separate. Bryant's traction can also be used for fractures of the femur.

Both lower extremities are incorporated in the traction setup even though only one extremity may be affected. Incorporating both extremities maintains immobilization and prevents the child from rotating around the affected extremity. This setup also facilitates care of the child, such as diaper or clothing changes, without interruption of the traction.

There are limits to the use of this traction in young children. The overhead position of the legs produces a strain on the circulation to the feet. Blood must be pumped against gravity to reach the suspended feet. When the child weighs more than 35 pounds, the amount of weight needed for traction could stretch the popliteal muscle. This would compress the blood vessels to the lower extremity and further impede circulation, eventually leading to the development of compartment syndrome.

The length of treatment in Bryant's traction depends on the purpose of the traction. The treatment duration for a child with DDH is usually 2 to 3 weeks, and the child may be cared for in the hospital or at home. To meet the child's developmental needs and to deal with the expected disruption of the family routine because of the child's limited mobility, a total plan of care is needed with DDH patients. When Bryant's traction is used for a child with a fracture, the child remains hospitalized for 2 to 3 weeks. Then, if x-rays show callus formation around the fracture site, the child is removed from the traction and placed in a body spica cast for another 3 to 9 weeks.

Mechanical Components

Angles: Both lower extremities are suspended vertically with the hips flexed at a 90 degree angle. The knees are slightly flexed at about 10 to 15 degrees. When Bryant's traction is used for divarication, the child's legs are gradually abducted over a period of several

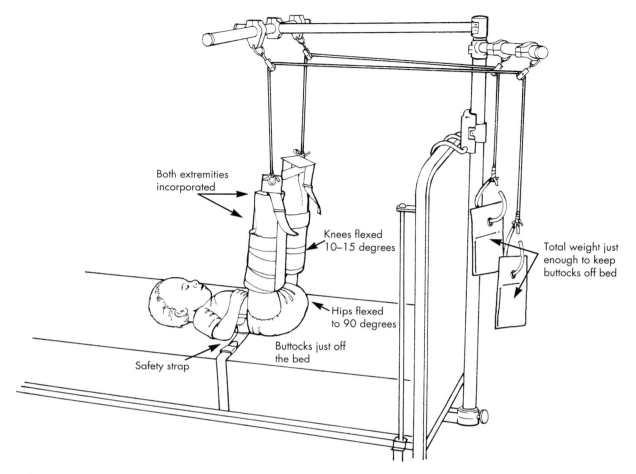

Both extremities incorporated

Knees flexed 10–15 degrees

Total weight just enough to keep buttocks off bed

Hips flexed to 90 degrees

Buttocks just off the bed

Safety strap

Figure 4-8 Bryant's traction is used with children under 3 years of age and weighing less than 35 pounds (15.9 kg) who have DDH.

days while the 90 degree flexion of the hips is maintained. This is accomplished by separating the pulleys on the overhead frame.

Weight. Enough weight is applied to keep the buttocks just above the bed. Usually less than half the weight of the child is sufficient. For example, if the child weighs 20 pounds, the weight needed to keep the buttocks just off the bed is 9 to 10 pounds (4.5 to 5 pounds [2.3 kg] per extremity).

Pulleys. A separate single pulley system is attached to each extremity. The overhead pulleys are connected at a point on the traction frame slightly distal to the buttocks.

Countertraction. The child's weight provides countertraction.

Applying Bryant's Traction

Before applying Bryant's traction, assess the skin. Because commercial adhesive strips are used most often, any redness, blistering, or break-down must be noted. Commercial boots are also available for Bryant's traction and can facilitate periodic removal for skin assessment. A physician applies the traction if the child is being treated for a fracture. With DDH, either the nurse or a trained family member may apply it.

Never remove Bryant's traction if the child is being treated for a fracture. For the child with DDH the physician will determine if the traction is to be removed and reapplied periodically. Some physicians allow the child to be out of traction for up to 30 minutes every 4 to 6 hours. If traction is to be removed and reapplied, provide specific instructions about what should be removed. In some cases only the weights should be removed, or the physician may want the elastic bandages unwrapped and rewrapped. Removing the tape strips applied to the skin is not recommended unless it is absolutely necessary; severe skin irritation can result.

To apply Bryant's traction, follow these instructions:

1. Place the child supine in the middle of the bed.
2. Pad the malleoli well.
3. Apply the foam strips to each side of the leg from just above the malleoli to just below the groin.
4. Make sure the knees are slightly flexed to prevent stretching the popliteal muscle and compressing the blood vessels.
5. Wrap each leg and strips with elastic bandages from the ankle to the thigh. Bandages should be wrinkle free and just snug enough to prevent slippage.
6. Make sure that the child can move the foot without causing skin irritation or constriction at the ankle.
7. Place a padded foot plate close enough to the foot that when the toes are extended they touch the plate.
8. Attach ropes to the foot plate and thread them through the pulley(s) attached to the frame.
9. Apply the appropriate weight (just enough to lift the child's buttocks off the bed).
10. Make sure that the weights hang freely and are not hanging over the child or where the child might be able to reach them. (See Figure 4-8.)
11. Apply a safety jacket or strap to keep the child in proper position and safely in the bed.

It may be helpful to have the child's parent or a guardian available to keep the child occupied and in the correct position while the traction is being applied. This may also help to decrease the child's anxiety.

Neurovascular dangers associated with skin traction include sloughing of the skin, ischemic necrosis, and compartment syndrome. The most common causes for these complications are tight bandages and hyperextension of the knees. The hyperextension places severe stress on the compartments, creating elevated compartment pressures. You must observe the child in Bryant's traction for appropriate alignment with the knees slightly flexed. Also, be aware that the child may develop compartment syndrome in either extremity; therefore neurovascular checks must include both extremities.

RELATED NURSING DIAGNOSES

Impaired physical mobility: Related to bedrest

Assessment	Rationale
Assess for proper positioning	Will facilitate healing process and reduction of dysplasia

Assessment	Rationale
Assess for safety of child and maintenance of T-strap or jacket	Keeps child in proper position to facilitate healing and decrease discomfort; may prevent accidents involving apparatus

Interventions

1. Encourage the parent to hold and cuddle the child.

2. If the traction cannot be removed for cuddling and holding, have the parent or guardian sit on a high stool next to the crib. Gently move the child over onto the lap of the adult. This may help the child and parent to bond while maintaining effective traction.

3. Do not allow the child who is permitted out of traction to stand or crawl.

4. Hold or place the child in a reclining seat similar to an infant car seat.

5. Develop an exercise program in collaboration with a specially trained occupational therapist.

Alteration in Skin Integrity: Related to bedrest and incontinence

Assessment	Rationale
Inspect skin at least every 2 to 3 hours	Potential skin problems may be recognized and treated immediately; wet diapers or other clothing or bed sheets **must** be changed in a timely manner, thereby decreasing risk of skin breakdown

Interventions

1. Inspect the skin at least every 2 to 3 hours.

2. Pay particular attention to the skin behind the knee and over the dorsum of the foot.

3. Check the skin of the back, especially the shoulder-blade area and back of the head. This area sometimes becomes wet when the child is incontinent.

4. Make sure that the pads and sheets are dry and unwrinkled.

5. Leave the diaper off for a short time to allow the skin to dry.

6. Remove and reapply the traction strips if they slip. When the child is being treated for a fracture, the physician must remove and reapply the strips. If the child is being treated for DDH, you may remove and reapply the strips.

7. Remove the tapes completely if there is any evidence of skin breakdown.

Self-Care Deficits: Related to bedrest and age

Assessment	Rationale
Assess for parent's willingness to perform activities of daily living (ADLs)	Allows for bonding of child and parent and also helps to decrease anxiety level for both parent and child
Assess for difficulty in swallowing	Because of position, child may be more prone to choking
Assess for developmental stage	If child is in process of being toilet trained, being in traction may be detrimental and this method of treatment may be reconsidered

Interventions

1. Bathe the child's buttocks and back after each voiding and bowel movement to maintain skin integrity.

2. Carefully feed the child and constantly observe because the child cannot sit up if a choking episode begins.

3. Give the child nutritional finger foods so he or she can participate in eating.

4. Avoid the serious problem of aspiration by feeding the child small mouthfuls, waiting, and holding the child's head when drinking.

5. Do not leave the child alone with the bottle.

6. Maintain the child's usual pattern of elimination. If the child is being toilet trained, interruption of this effort may have long-term effects. This developmental issue should be addressed by the physician, the parents, and the nurses caring for the child in an effort to provide consistency in treatment.

Increased Risk of Neurovascular Dysfunction: Related to traction apparatus and position

Assessment	Rationale
Assess for pulses, color, and temperature of extremity	Decreased or absent pulses, blue or white color, and coolness of extremity may indicate vascular compromise
Assess for movement and sensation of lower extremities	Decreased movement or sensation may indicate neurological problem; if gently moving foot causes obvious increase in pain, may indicate compartment syndrome

Interventions

1. Notify the physician immediately if neurovascular impairment is suspected.

2. Loosen the dressings, reduce the traction, and, if necessary, move the legs down from the suspended position until circulation is restored. (If the child is being treated for a fracture, this must be done by the physician.) After circulation is restored, rewrap the legs with the elastic wrap, using less tension. Then reestablish the traction.

3. Investigate any evidence of pain. Because the child may not be able to verbalize discomfort, you must be aware of any change in the child's temperament or of the child's crying for no apparent reason.

Impaired Gas Exchange: Related to position and bedrest

Assessment	Rationale
Assess for breath sounds, respirations, and temperature	Being in dependent position may increase risk of pneumonia and aspiration

Interventions

1. Treat any symptoms of upper respiratory infection immediately.

2. Monitor vital signs.

3. Feed the child carefully to avoid aspiration.

4. **Never** leave the child unattended.

Ineffective coping: Related to bedrest and hospitalization

Assessment	Rationale
Assess for normal developmental stages	Treatment in traction may interrupt normal developmental process
Assess child's support systems	Including child's siblings is necessary for psychosocial development

Interventions

1. Institute a plan to allow for the continuation of normal developmental processes. Include the child's parents, a pediatric occupational therapist, a child life specialist, a clinical nurse specialist, and the physician. Make the plan as soon as possible and communicate it to all health professionals and others who come in contact with the child. The child must be treated consistently by all persons encountered during the treatment period.

2. Include the child's siblings in the plan; they are an important part of the child's psychosocial development. For the child being treated for DDH, the 30-minute release from traction every 4 hours is an ideal time for continued contact with siblings or other children and adults.

CARE GUIDE
BUCK'S AND RUSSELL'S TRACTION

The following information should be used in conjunction with the information found in the general traction management guide (Chapter 3).

MECHANICAL COMPONENTS

1. Weight . . . .

   Buck's traction
   a. Should not exceed 8 pounds

   Russell's traction
   a. Should not exceed 4 to 5 pounds

2. Pulleys . . . .

   Buck's traction
   a. One-pulley system in straight line

   Russell's traction
   a. Double-pulley system at foot
   b. Single-pulley system at knee

3. Ropes . . . .

   a. See general traction management guide (Chapter 3)

4. Countertraction . . . .

   a. Foot of bed elevated about 6 inches

5. Angles . . . .

   Buck's traction
   a. Pull is in straight line
   b. Flat pillow or bath blanket **only** to keep pressure off heel

   Russell's traction
   a. Angle between thigh and mattress is 20 degrees
   b. Leg is supported on pillows to maintain angle

6. Bed . . . . a. See general traction management guide (Chapter 3)

7. Trapeze . . . . a. See general traction management guide (Chapter 3)

8. Traction boot . . . .
   a. Boot is appropriate size
   b. Securely in place
   c. Foot plate not leaning against pulley
   d. Heel is appropriately placed in boot
   e. Foot is flat against bottom
   f. Boot sides are overlapped
   g. Velcro straps attached using moderate tension
   h. No pressure on popliteal space
   h. No pressure on popliteal space
   i. Boot is applied to bare leg

9. Adhesive straps . . . .
   a. Preapplication assessment completed:
      (1) Adequate neurovascular status
      (2) No abrasions
      (3) No open areas
      (4) No infections
      (5) No reddened areas
      (6) No allergies
   b. Extremity shaved if necessary
   c. Traction strips extend from malleolus to just below fibular head
   d. Malleolus and fibular head well padded
   e. Elastic bandage applied
      (1) Foot included
      (2) Wrapped to just below knee
      (3) Applied with even tension
   f. Foot piece wide enough to prevent pressure on side of foot

10. Sling (Russell's only) . . . .
   a. Supports leg at knee
   b. No wrinkles
   c. No irritation in popliteal space
   d. No pressure on fibular head

PATIENT ALIGNMENT

a. Patient is straight in bed
b. Affected leg supported appropriately
c. Buck's: Extremity is straight
   Russell's: Hip and knee flexed
d. All essential items within reach of patient
e. Turn patient side to side using pillows to support extremity
f. **Get help when necessary**

SKIN INTEGRITY

a. See general traction management guide (Chapter 3)
b. Check knee support of Russell's traction
   (1) No pressure on popliteal space
   (2) No pressure on fibular head
   (3) No irritation in popliteal space
c. Check affected extremity in boot
   (1) Proper fit
   (2) Proper heel placement
   (3) No pressure on heel
   (4) No pressure on malleoli
   (5) No pressure on dorsum of foot
d. Check affected extremity in strips (see above)

▼

CARE GUIDE
BRYANT'S TRACTION

The following information should be used in conjunction with the information found in the general traction management guide (Chapter 3).

MECHANICAL COMPONENTS

1. Weights . . . .
   a. Prescribed amount by doctor; usually half the weight of child, with half applied to each leg; should be sufficient to allow buttocks to be barely off mattress

2. Pulleys . . . .
   a. Single separate pulley system for each leg; child should be placed in bed so pulleys are slightly distal to buttocks
   b. An additional crossbar and pulley are used to position weights away from child
   c. Bed frame supports traction apparatus and should be checked for tightness of all knobs securing apparatus to bed
   d. Knots in ropes should be at least 12 inches from pulley

3. Ropes . . . .
   a. Freely movable in pulley groove
   b. Knots secured with tape
   c. No kinks or fraying
   d. Located so child cannot move to reach ropes
   e. No toys or plants attached to ropes

4. Countertraction . . . .
   a. Countertraction is provided by weight of child; space between buttock and mattress should be barely enough to slide hand under buttocks

5. Angles . . . .

a. Legs at 90 degree angle to hip
b. Knees must be slightly flexed (10 to 15 degrees)
c. Buttocks should be off bed no more than width of finger
d. Foot plate positioned so extended toes can touch it

6. Bed . . . .

a. Crib with side rails is recommended; side rails should be up at all times, except when providing care
b. Firm mattress with moisture barrier is recommended

PATIENT ALIGNMENT

a. Child should be straight in bed with pulley on overhead frame placed just distal to buttocks
b. Restraint may be necessary for safety of child and to assure proper application of traction
   (1) Consult pediatric texts and/or clinical specialists for assistance in restraining child in traction
   (2) Sling restraint over pelvic area is most frequently used method
   (3) Restraint must be applied so as not to increase effect of countertraction
c. Legs should be positioned so knees are flexed at 10-to-15-degree angle; hyperextension can cause serious complications
d. Hips should be flexed at 90-degree angle
   (1) Feet should be slightly extended but able to touch plate
   (2) Should not press against footplate or be hyperextended
e. If permitted by physician, child can be taken out of traction
   (1) To move child with traction apparatus in place, use chair or stool that is same height as mattress

PATIENT ALIGNMENT–cont'd

      (2) While sitting on stool, carefully slide child onto your lap, being sure that traction line is not interrupted

      (3) If traction is being used for fracture, child should **not** be moved

MAINTENANCE OF SKIN INTEGRITY

1. Check pressure points . . . .
   a. Sacrum, coccyx, spine, shoulder blades, back of head, ears
   b. Any point where traction wrap is near bony prominence (e.g., head of tibia, malleolus at ankle, dorsum of foot, and Achilles tendon)
   c. Diaper area and back (for wetness)

EVALUATION OF AFFECTED EXTREMITIES

1. Alteration in tissue perfusion . . . .
   a. Check pulses in dorsum of foot and color and warmth of each foot; also check capillary filling and ability to move toes
   b. Make note of any change in behavior, especially if child appears to be in pain

NURSING CARE

1. Alteration in gas exchange . . . .
   a. Because of child's dependent position, upper respiratory tract must be assessed for any signs of infection or congestion

2. Alteration in nutritional status . . . .
   a. Schedule times out of traction to coincide with meals

3. Alteration in elimination . . . .
   a. Bowel patterns should be monitored

4. Developmental needs . . . .
   a. Child's normal developmental needs must be addressed, and consultation with appropriate professionals is recommended

5. Ineffective coping by parents or other caregiver . . . .

    a. Explain all procedures, especially when there is change in plan; for example, if child needs restraint, give parents full explanation

    b. Allow parents to participate in care plan as much as possible

    c. Encourage normal patterns of growth and development for child and other members of family, especially if there are siblings

DISCHARGE PLANNING

1. Preparing child for home . . . .

    a. Full assessment of needs of child and family should be done as early in treatment as possible, ideally as soon as it is determined that child can be cared for in home setting

    b. Allow parents to provide care for period of 8 to 24 hours under supervision of hospital staff

    c. Make referral to home care nursing agency for follow-up teaching and monitoring

    d. Order all necessary traction equipment from home medical equipment and services company; make sure that equipment is delivered and set up at home before patient is discharged

5 Skeletal Traction to the Lower Extremity and Hip

Skeletal traction involves applying a pulling force directly to the bony skeleton by using pins or wires through the bone distal to the fracture or tongs embedded within the skull. (See Chapter 2.)

Balanced-Suspension Traction

Skeletal traction with balanced suspension is commonly used to treat fractures of the femur, hip, acetabulum, and pelvis. Pins are usually inserted into the proximal tibia or distal femur. However, if surgery is anticipated, the distal femur is avoided because the surgical wound's chances of becoming infected increase if the pin site becomes infected.

After the pin is inserted (using aseptic technique usually in the operating room), the leg is placed in a splint, usually a Thomas or Harris splint, and then affixed with a Pearson attachment. The splint and Pearson attachment are suspended and balanced from the overhead frame by a system of weights and pulleys. The leg and splint constitute one unit; only the hip moves. No motion occurs at the fracture site, so proper alignment is maintained. A **pin holder** or horseshoe traction bow is then attached to the pin. The rope is fastened to the holder, runs through a system of

pulleys, and then is affixed to the weight holder or bag at the end of the bed (Fig. 5-1).

Mechanical Components

Angles. The physician determines the best position of the lower extremity to align the distal fragment of the bone with the proximal fragment. Overriding of the fragments or severe muscle spasm may hamper this initially. After the position has been determined, the weights are applied to achieve anatomical position of the fracture fragments. Once the determined position is obtained, it must be maintained even though the angles may appear somewhat exaggerated.

Weights. The average initial weight on the lower extremity is 10 to 25 pounds for an adult. The physician determines the weight needed based on each patient's needs. Factors to consider include the type and position of the fracture and the age, weight, and stature of the patient. X-rays are taken to determine and maintain the necessary amount of weight for repair of the fracture.

Pulleys. Skeletal traction uses a single-pulley system (straight-line traction) separate from the system that suspends the Thomas splint and Pearson attachment. The amount of traction force used equals the weight applied.

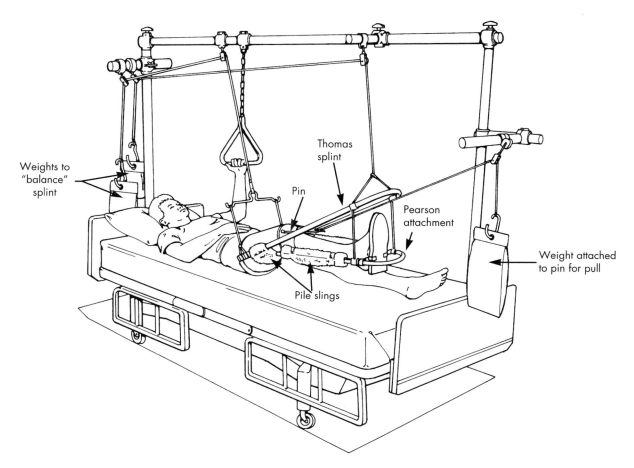

Figure 5-1 Balanced-suspension traction to the lower extremity. This type of traction uses one pulley for traction; therefore the amount of weight equals the amount of pull.

Countertraction. Countertraction can be achieved by elevating the foot of the bed approximately 6 inches, by stringing weights from the splint to the head of the bed, or by using the patient's own body weight.

Thomas Splint

One side of a Thomas splint is shorter than the other. The short side is placed on the inner as-

pect of the thigh. The half ring under the thigh is attached by a swivel so the splint may be used for either leg. The half ring is placed under the thigh to avoid unnecessary pressure on the femoral artery and nerve. Because it is movable, the half ring may flatten out as the patient slides down in bed. This causes the patient to sit on the edge of the ring, causing discomfort and compromising skin integrity. The half ring must always be at a right angle to the frame. (To restore the ring to a right angle, have the patient lift slightly, grasp the ring, and pull it forward.)

The pile slings, stretched across the splint, support the leg. They should be securely attached with serrated traction clips. Safety pins should not be used because they tend to spring open and increase the risk of injury to the patient and caregiver. Enough slings and clips must be used to provide even support of the extremity. To decrease the risk of skin breakdown, the bed sheet must be taut and wrinkle free. The foot piece is placed where it can support the foot in a neutral position. Enough space should be provided to allow some movement of the foot for exercise and to decrease the risk of skin breakdown, especially over the metatarsal heads.

Position of the Leg in the Splint

The placement of the leg in the splint remains the same regardless of the angles of flexion and the amount of abduction used. When the leg is properly seated in the splint, the ring lies under the thigh just distal to the gluteal fold. The Pearson attachment is secured to the Thomas splint where it coincides with the axis of movement of the knee. The angle of the knee is maintained by tying a rope to the end of the Pearson attachment and extending it to the end of the Thomas splint. The Pearson attachment may be suspended by its own pulley system when movement of the knee is desirable, as with fracture of the tibial plateau. Usually the lower leg is parallel to the mattress.

Boehler-Braun Frame (Calcaneus Site)

For open (compound) fractures of the tibia with severe soft tissue damage, unstable tibial fractures, or severe ankle fractures, skeletal traction with a pin or wire placed through the calcaneus is used. It requires a special apparatus called the Boehler-Braun frame, which rests on the bed and supports the leg in a fixed position. The traction is applied directly through the pulley on the frame. Because the traction is self-contained and independent of the bed, it may be used if the patient must be transported (Fig. 5-2).

Mechanical Components

Angles. The leg is supported with the hip and knee each flexed about 45 degrees. This flexed position serves two purposes: (1) The strong muscles of the lower leg originate above the knee joint. By keeping the knee flexed, the pull of these muscles is minimized and therefore the risk of displacing fracture fragments is decreased. (2) The release of the natural pull of the muscles permits the fracture's position to be maintained with a small amount of traction weight. Keeping the leg supported on pile slings stretched across the frame (as in balanced suspension) and using an adequate number of slings and clips will decrease the risk of posterior angulation of the fracture secondary to gravity.

Weights. The amount of weight rarely exceeds 5 pounds because the calcaneus is cancellous bone and cannot withstand a great amount of pull. The wire used is also usually of a smaller diameter. Large amounts of weight may cause bowing of the pin or actual cutting of the bone.

Pulleys. The Boehler-Braun frame incorporates a single-pulley system.

Countertraction. Countertraction is provided by the thigh resting against the inclined plane of the frame.

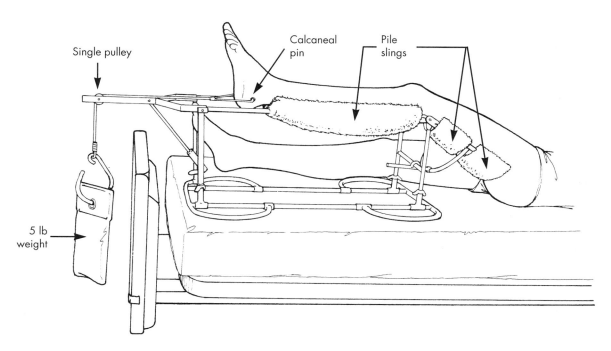

Figure 5-2   The Boehler-Braun frame (calcaneus site).

Care of the Patient in Skeletal Traction

Your concerns as a nurse when caring for a patient in skeletal traction include skin integrity, self-care deficits, pain, elimination, immobility, and the risk of neurological and vascular impairment. Also you must manage the patient's mechanical apparatus so optimum benefits will result:

1. Check daily to ensure that the bed frame is securely fastened to the bed and all cross bars and pulleys are secure.
2. Observe the traction ropes carefully for weakening, especially when large amounts of weight are used over long periods. The rope can break without obvious signs of fraying. To prevent abrupt and painful interruption of the traction, attach a safety line by tying an additional rope alongside the traction rope. If the traction rope breaks, the second rope can maintain the traction. This decreases the risk of a painful jolt or loss of the fracture's position. Nylon rope may also be used; it has a lower incidence of fraying and breaking.
3. To prevent slipping, tape all ends of the rope that are tied to either the frame or the weight holder.
4. **Do not reuse traction rope.** Even though the integrity of the rope appears intact, the constant stress of the weights may have weakened the fibers to the point that they will no longer support additional weight.

5. Attach the trapeze to the traction bed frame so the bar hangs slightly anterior to the patient's shoulders.
6. Adjust the length of the trapeze so that when the patient is grasping the bar the elbows are flexed approximately 20 degrees.

Maintaining Proper Position of the Patient

1. The patient must be lying straight in bed. Leaning to one side may change the angle set by the physician and thus interfere with the line of pull.
2. Position the patient in the middle of the bed so that when the head of the bed is elevated (if permitted) the hips rest at the break in the mattress.
3. Avoid elevating the head of the bed more than 35 degrees except for short periods when the patient is eating and bathing. Elevating above this level may cause the patient to slide down in the bed and interfere with the effectiveness of traction.

Positioning the Extremity

1. Keep the extremity aligned as established by the physician.
2. Check to see that the half ring of the Thomas splint is kept at a right angle to the splint and just distal to the gluteal fold so as to provide proper support and reduce the chance of skin breakdown.
3. Avoid pressure in the perineal area.
4. Check to see that the pile slings on which the extremity is lying provide equal support to the entire extremity.
5. Check the pile slings for soiling. If the slings must be changed, remove and replace them one at a time so as to maintain uninterrupted support of the extremity.
6. The cover of the half ring is frequently made of nonporous padding material that can be wiped clean with soap and water. If soiling is excessive, the lining may be removed and replaced. (See manufacturer's recommendations.)
7. Fasten the foot piece to the Pearson attachment so the foot is supported in a neutral position, allowing enough room for the patient to plantarflex the foot. If the sling surrounding the foot piece is too tight, it may cause pressure on the metatarsal heads.

Moving the Patient

The patient can be lifted for skin care, linen changes, and bedpan use. Throughout the lifting procedure the goal is to maintain effective traction and cause the patient the least amount of discomfort. The following guidelines help to accomplish this:

1. To move the patient comfortably, describe the adjustments you will be making so that the patient can cooperate. **Explain what you are going to do before you do it.**
2. Have the patient assist as much as possible.
3. Use a firm, steady motion when moving or adjusting the extremity in traction. This approach helps to minimize muscle spasm and decrease discomfort.
4. When lifting or moving the patient for back care, place your hands under the patient from the unaffected side to avoid direct handling of the fracture area.
5. If the patient is allowed to have and can use a trapeze, it may help him or her to move in bed more easily. Instruct the patient to grab the trapeze bar, bend the knee of the unaffected leg, and push down with the foot while pulling up on the bar.
6. Avoid bumping the bed or traction apparatus. Sudden movements may cause pain and spasm.

7. When both lower extremities are in traction, assistance in lifting is usually required for back care, bedpan change, and linen changes. Use at least two people, taking into consideration the patient's ability to assist. Position one person on each side of the bed, lifting the patient using open-palmed hands. Avoid contact with the fracture site.

RELATED NURSING DIAGNOSES

Impaired Physical Mobility: Related to prolonged bedrest

Assessment	Rationale
Assess all bony prominences	Helps to maintain skin integrity
Assess patient's ability to move extremities	May be used as basis for establishing exercise program

Interventions

1. Establish a comprehensive exercise program to maintain muscle mass, strength, and tone, to maintain full range of motion of the joints, and to promote circulation in the affected extremities.

2. Plan exercises within the therapeutic limits of the traction, the extent of the patient's injuries, and the patient's ability to perform them. (See Chapter 4.)

3. Establish the exercise program with assistance of the physical and occupational therapists. Exercises for the affected extremity in a balanced suspension frame include the following:

   a. Gluteal and quadriceps setting (isometric) exercises.

   b. Ankle circling. Remove the pile sling foot support to allow full circling, which includes dorsiflexion, plantarflexion, and circumduction. Ankle circling may be contraindicated in patients using the Boehler-Braun frame because of the placement of the pin. However, dorsiflexion and plantarflexion may be allowed.

   c. If the physician orders movement of the knee of the affected extremity, this is accomplished by securing the Pearson attachment to its own system of weights and pulleys and then attaching a handle to the rope. The patient can flex and extend the knee by pulling on the rope.

Alteration in Skin Integrity: Related to immobility

Assessment	Rationale
Assess skin integrity on admission to hospital	May need to change treatment plan if open areas are present or if skin integrity is otherwise questionable
Assess patient's complaints of discomfort	May indicate area of concern that is not evident on initial examination (e.g., a deep bruise)
Assess for swelling of extremity	To prevent development of compartment syndrome; also fracture of large bone (femur) may be accompanied by excessive bleeding into surrounding soft tissues, resulting in extremely swollen extremity and putting pressure on compartments

Assessment	Rationale
Assess nutritional status and hydration	Patient who is malnourished or dehydrated is at increased risk of skin breakdown secondary to depleted protein stores and fluid deficiency
Assess mental status	Patient who is confused or agitated may be more prone to skin breakdown because of excessive movement; also may be prone to incontinence and noncompliance

Interventions

1. Make sure the ring of the traction frame is always in contact with the posterior thigh. Adjust the amount of weight applied to suspend the frame to accomplish this. If the frame does not lift when the patient lifts, more weight may be needed. If the frame is pressing into the posterior thigh and causing discomfort, a weight adjustment may be necessary. These adjustments can be made only on order of the physician.

2. The object of balanced-suspension traction is to allow the patient to lift and move yet maintain the leg in the predetermined position. **Do not** turn the patient from side to side. Turning causes severe discomfort, allows pins to slip or injure the other extremity, and increases the chance of rendering the traction ineffective. Give back care by lifting the patient or, preferably, by instructing the patient to lift himself or herself. Often, to protect both patient and personnel, more than one person is needed for lifting. If the traction is effective and properly balanced, the patient will not experience severe pain when moving. Never lift traction weights when moving or lifting the patient.

3. On rare occasions with the multiple-trauma patient (e.g., combined cervical traction and balanced-suspension traction), lifting may be contraindicated. In this situation the patient can be turned side to side (providing the injuries are stable and the physician has ordered turning), but no more than 20 to 30 degrees or only enough to facilitate inspection and massage of the buttocks and back. Make sure that the splint and leg are supported so they act as one unit. Also, if the patient has a cervical fracture, the head and neck must be adequately supported. Turning the patient requires two people on the side to which the patient is being turned. When turning is complete, be sure that the splint and leg are properly repositioned.

For the patient in the Boehler-Braun frame, the following points should be noted:

- To facilitate bed changes, apply one sheet from the head of the bed down to the frame, and the other under the frame to the bottom of the bed. This will eliminate the need to move the frame at every bed change.
- For back care, turn the patient toward the affected side.
- Keep the heel of the affected extremity free of pressure; it should not rest on the pile sling covering the frame. Pad the Achilles tendon area well (an extra-pile sling is recommended), massage the heel frequently, and observe for signs of pressure or irritation.

Pain: Related to injury

Assessment	Rationale
Assess for signs and symptoms of pain or discomfort	May indicate that treatment is not appropriate or that traction is not properly applied

Assessment	Rationale
Assess for signs and symptoms of pain or discomfort	Indicates need to offer or administer analgesics May indicate possible complications (e.g., thrombophlebitis)

Interventions

1. Carefully examine the patient and traction apparatus to determine the cause of discomfort. If the pain is due to interruption of the traction or to muscle spasm, it may be alleviated by reestablishment of the traction or a minor adjustment in the equipment.

2. Make sure that the patient is in proper alignment.

3. Administer analgesics and muscle relaxants as ordered.

4. Institute other modalities to help decrease discomfort. Examples include diversional activities, meditation, and guided imagery.

Pin Site Care

The insertion and exit sites of the pin or wire used in skeletal traction require observation and daily care. Procedures and protocols may differ in each institution, and individual care may be ordered according to physician preference.

Usually the sites are cleaned daily with an antiseptic solution and covered with a sterile gauze cut to fit around the pin next to the skin. General points to consider are as follows:

- Observe the pin sites for signs of infection. Note any redness, elevated temperature (both of the surrounding skin and of the body), edema of the area, increased pain at the pin sites, prolonged serosanguineous drainage, or purulent drainage.

- Keep the area clean according to orders.

- A pin site infection can lead to a more serious disorder because the pin acts as a direct link from the external environment to the bone. Contamination may cause a major infection (osteomyelitis) requiring removal of the pin and the possibility of long-term complications.

- Slight serous oozing at the pin site is to be expected, especially for the first 2 to 3 days, but eventually decreases. However, motion between the pin and the bone can result in the formation of excess serous drainage. If this is allowed to collect, it can become a site for infection.

- Prevent crusting around the pin site; this can block adequate drainage of the serous fluid and trap bacteria. Gently remove the crusting using a sterile cotton-tipped swab dipped in a cleansing solution such as hydrogen peroxide and normal saline (50/50). Starting at the site, use a gentle rolling motion to lift the crusts away from the site. Avoid digging into the pin site. Once the crusts have been removed, apply an antibacterial solution such as an iodine preparation, according to hospital and/or physician preference.

- Avoid tenting of the skin at the pin site (stretching of skin around the pin, with adherence to the pin creating a tentlike appearance), because this can interfere with adequate drainage. The physician may elect to make a sterile surgical incision when the pin is inserted, which will help to prevent the skin from adhering to the pin and thus compromising adequate drainage.

- To prevent infection, instruct the patient not to touch the area surrounding the pin site.

- Watch for migration of the pin, which can cause pressure on the skin (from the bow) and subsequent skin breakdown if it is not relieved.
- If the pin care method used involves wrapping sterile stretch gauze around the pin and leaving it in place (e.g., a figure-eight dressing around the pin), wrapping may not prevent the pin from moving. The gauze itself can cause skin breakdown as the bow pushes against the skin.
- Place a cork, adhesive tape, rubber stopper, or commercially available product over the protruding sharp ends of the pin or wire so they do not scratch or otherwise harm the patient or caregiver.

Increased Risk of Neurovascular Dysfunction: Related to injury or immobility

Ongoing assessment of the patient's neurological status and circulation to the extremity is an integral part of the nursing management of patients in traction. It is especially important for patients in skeletal traction, because the nerves or vessels can be impaired by placement of the pin or wire or can be compressed by the traction apparatus. Also, because some injuries requiring skeletal traction are accompanied by excessive blood loss, monitoring of these parameters is mandatory.

To assess neurological status, follow these directions:

- Ascertain if the patient is experiencing any pain, numbness, tingling, or loss of sensation by lightly touching the extremity with your hand or an open paper clip, being careful not to break the skin. Causing a break in the skin may increase the risk of infection.
- Check for continued motor function. Ask the patient to move the toes of both feet.
- Ascertain if the patient can feel gentle pressure exerted on a point distal to (below) the injury or traction application site.
- Document and notify the physician immediately of any deficit in these areas.

To assess circulatory status, do the following:

- Check for the presence and quality of pulses distal to (below) the injury or traction application site.
- Assess capillary filling: Use the blanching sign, which evaluates arterial return. Gently pinch the skin or nail bed of the affected extremity below the injury or traction application site. The nail bed or skin should "blanch" or turn white. However, as soon as the pressure of the pinch is eliminated, the area should return to its normal pink color. The rapidity with which this occurs demonstrates the presence or absence of capillary refill. If the skin does not return to its normal color within 2 to 4 seconds, suspect damage to the arterial circulation. Report and document these findings immediately. Poor capillary filling may indicate that the traction apparatus is applied too tightly or incorrectly or that there is an underlying injury to the vascular system.
- Observe for swelling, warmth, and color. Some residual swelling from the original injury may exist, but the extremity should be warm to the touch and the color should be about the same as that of the unaffected extremity. If the extremity is cold to the touch, has a whitish blue appearance, or has whitish blue nail beds, vascular integrity may be compromised.

Report and document these findings immediately.

- Ascertain if motion of the digits of the affected extremity greatly increases pain. Gently move the toes of the extremity; if the patient complains of extreme pain, beyond what is normal or expected, compartment syndrome, a potentially limb-threatening condition, may be present. This results from compression of the nerves and vessels contained within the compartments of the extremity. The syndrome is explained in greater detail in Chapter 9.

Impaired Gas Exchange: Related to bedrest

Assessment	Rationale
Assess respiratory status; auscultate lungs	Decrease breath sounds, rales or rhonchi, or wheezing may indicate hypostatic pneumonia
Assess vital signs, including temperature, pulse, and respirations	Hypostatic pneumonia may develop: signs include elevated temperature, congestion, increased respiratory rate, dyspnea, and cyanosis

Interventions

1. Use caution in administering drugs that may decrease the rate and depth of lung expansion and depress the cough reflex.

2. Observe the patient for signs and symptoms associated with hypostatic pneumonia (i.e., shortness of breath, elevated temperature, dyspnea, cyanosis, congestion, lethargy).

3. Instruct the patient in the use of respiratory aid procedures such as incentive spirometry, coughing, and deep breathing. These will help the patient to inhale deeply.

4. Do not allow the patient to smoke.

CARE GUIDE
BALANCED-SUSPENSION TRACTION

The following information should be used in conjunction with the information found in the general traction management guide (Chapter 3).

MECHANICAL COMPONENTS

1. Weights . . . .
   a. Prescribed amount by physician
   b. Securely attached
   c. Hanging freely
      (1) Not caught on bed
      (2) Not caught on frame
      (3) Not on floor
      (4) Not hanging over patient
   d. At least 12 inches from pulley

2. Pulleys . . . .
   a. Securely attached to bed frame
   b. Wheels move freely

3. Ropes . . . .
   a. In groove of pulley
   b. Freely movable
   c. No fraying
   d. No kinks or unnecessary knots
   e. Knots taped to prevent slipping
   f. Safety ropes in place

4. Countertraction . . . .
   a. Countertraction provided by
      (1) 6-inch shock blocks under foot of bed
      (2) Trendelenburg position

5. Bed . . . .
   a. Firm mattress
   b. Bed boards if applicable
   c. Side rails
   d. Frame securely attached to bed
   e. Crossbars securely attached to frame (check daily)

6. Trapeze . . . .
   - a. Securely attached to frame
   - b. Hangs so patient's elbows are flexed 20 degrees
   - c. Attached slightly anterior to level of patient's shoulders

PATIENT ALIGNMENT

1. Traction pull . . . .
   - a. Traction apparatus freely movable but not impinging on bed frame or resting against pulleys
   - b. Patient straight in bed with buttocks positioned at break of mattress
   - c. Balanced-suspension frame moves with patient when patient lifts; ring remains in contact with posterior thigh
   - d. All necessary items are within reach of patient
   - e. Head of bed elevated no more than 35 degrees

2. Leg in Thomas splint with Pearson attachment . . . .
   - a. Should be straight in frame
   - b. Slings clean and equally taut
   - c. Slings adequate in number to give full support
   - d. Half ring maintained at right angle to Thomas splint
   - e. Half ring padding clean and in place
   - f. Foot support allows for adequate movement of foot

3. Provision of comfort when moving patient
   - a. Explain procedure to patient
   - b. Teach patient how to use trapeze
   - c. Use firm and steady motion; avoid bumping or jarring bed or traction apparatus
   - d. **Get help when necessary**

MAINTENANCE OF SKIN INTEGRITY

1. Check pressure points . . . .
   a. General: sacrum, heels, coccyx, trochanters, spine, scapulae
   b. Specific to Thomas splint: groin, ischium, perineum, genitalia
   c. Lower extremity: Achilles tendon, metatarsals, malleoli, head of fibula

2. Check for increased risk of skin breakdown
   a. See general traction management guide (Chapter 3)

3. Adjunct equipment to decrease risk of skin breakdown . . . .
   a. Special mattress or mattress covers
      (1) Egg crate
      (2) Water
      (3) Air
   b. Protectors for heels and/or elbows
   c. Pillow supports
   d. Sheepskin
   e. Therapeutic bed

EVALUATION OF AFFECTED EXTREMITY

1. Alteration in tissue perfusion (circulation)
   a. Check pulses distal to injury or traction site
   b. Check capillary filling (normal 2 to 4 seconds)
   c. Observe for
      (1) Warmth
      (2) Color
      (3) Swelling
      (4) Increased size of thigh circumference
      (5) Compare to unaffected extremity
      (6) Check for Homan's sign

2. Potential for pin site infection . . . .
   a. Check pin site for redness, warmth, edema, pain, prolonged drainage, purulent drainage, tenting
   b. Check to see that pin site is clean and free of encrustation
   c. Check for migration of pin

        d. Provide prescribed pin site care

        e. Instruct patient not to touch area around pin site

3. Alteration in neurological status . . . .   a. Check for motion of extremity
          (1) Ability to move toes
          (2) Ability to dorsiflex foot
        b. Check for sensation
          (1) Pressure and touch
          (2) Pain
          (3) Numbness
          (4) Tingling

NURSING CARE

1. Alteration in gas exchange . . . .   a. Have patient cough and deep breathe
        b. Have patient demonstrate correct use of incentive spirometry
        c. Suction and oxygen apparatus available if necessary

2. Alteration in nutritional status . . . .   a. Patient eats well-balanced diet
        b. Patient is properly positioned for meals (head of bed may be elevated up to 35 degrees)
        c. Food is presented so patient can manage to feed self (i.e., meat is cut, containers opened, finger foods provided)
        d. Patient drinks adequate fluids
        e. Food supplements provided as necessary

3. Alteration in elimination . . . .   a. Encourage fluids
        b. Check for urinary retention and institute appropriate nursing measures
        c. Establish pattern for elimination
          (1) Offer bedpan on regular schedule
          (2) Use fracture pan
          (3) Provide privacy

d. Encourage natural laxative foods and fluids

e. Check for constipation and institute appropriate nursing measures

4. Alteration in activity and exercise . . . .

a. Instruct patient in bed exercise program and reasons for it

b. Observe patient for follow-through on exercise schedule

c. Encourage self-care within limits of ability

5. Ineffective coping . . . .

a. Explain procedures and rationale for treatment to patient

b. Allow patient to verbalize

c. Answer patient's questions honestly (or refer to appropriate person)

d. Encourage involvement of family and friends

e. Provide diversional activities

f. Investigate home and family situation to assess need for intervention (discharge planning)

g. Make referrals to appropriate support services

h. Schedule team conferences with all disciplines involved in care; revise plan of care as needed

i. Provide for patient's spiritual needs

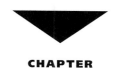

Skin and Skeletal Traction to the Upper Extremity

Traction to the upper extremity may be applied by either the skin or the skeletal approach depending on where the fracture is, the desired therapeutic effect, the associated injuries, and the physician's preference. Upper extremity traction is used to immobilize supracondylar fractures and dislocations of the elbow, humerus, and shoulder. The traction pull is always exerted on the humerus; the forearm is held in suspension only.

Three types of traction to the upper extremity are sidearm, Dunlop's, and overhead 90-90. Sidearm traction and Dunlop's traction are usually applied to the skin, although sidearm traction can be applied using a skeletal pin through the olecranon process. Overhead 90-90 traction is applied using a skeletal pin.

Sidearm Traction

Sidearm traction involves the application of lateral-longitudinal traction to the humerus. As already stated, it may be applied by the skin or skeletal method. This type of traction usually employs a special frame that attaches to the bed frame and allows the head of the bed to be elevated without disrupting the angles and pull of the traction. If the special frame is not used, the head of the bed must remain flat (Fig. 6-1).

The skin application of sidearm traction is accomplished by using adhesive straps wrapped with elastic bandages. There are two separate skin applications: one to the humerus (to apply longitudinal traction) and one to the forearm (to hold the arm in a lateral position). Application to the forearm provides for suspension of the arm in the sidearm position.

The major indication for skin application of sidearm traction is the treatment of fractures or dislocations not requiring large amounts of weight or long periods of immobilization. It may also be used in the treatment of children.

The skeletal and skin application of sidearm traction may be combined by using a pin through the olecranon process of the ulna for the longitudinal pull and skin traction applied to the forearm for suspension of the arm. The pin used for the skeletal application is usually of a small diameter (e.g., a Kirschner wire).

Mechanical Components

Angles. The pulling force is applied to the humerus in a lateral-longitudinal line. The traction force pulls longitudinally on the humerus. The shoulder is abducted 90 degrees from the body and is externally rotated as ordered by the physician. The elbow is flexed 90 degrees and is suspended perpendicular to the bed.

55

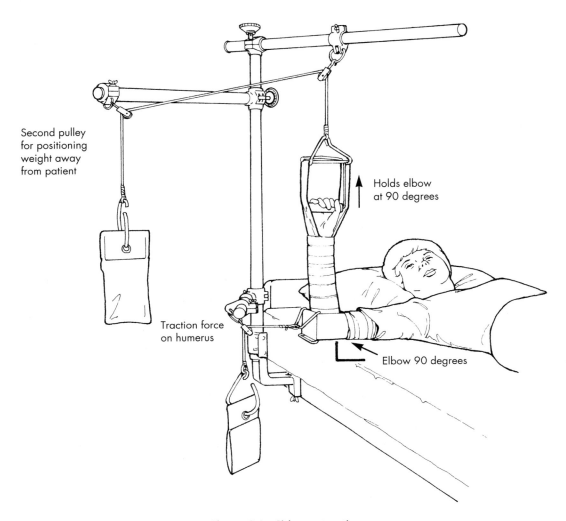

Second pulley
for positioning
weight away
from patient

Holds elbow
at 90 degrees

Traction force
on humerus

Elbow 90 degrees

Figure 6-1 Sidearm traction.

Weight. There are two sets of weights in sidearm traction. One exerts a pulling force on the humerus and one holds the elbow at a 90-degree angle, thus suspending the arm. The sidearm apparatus uses only enough weight to hold the arm in a lateral position so the traction pull is in a straight line. The amount of weight applied depends on the method of application. If skin traction is used, no more than

3 pounds should be used for each component. If skeletal traction is applied, the amount of weight applied to the skeletal pin should not exceed 10 pounds.

Pulleys. Sidearm traction uses two single-pulley systems, one for the longitudinal pull and one for suspension of the forearm. In Figure 6-1 two pulleys are used for suspension of the forearm. This prevents the weights from hang-

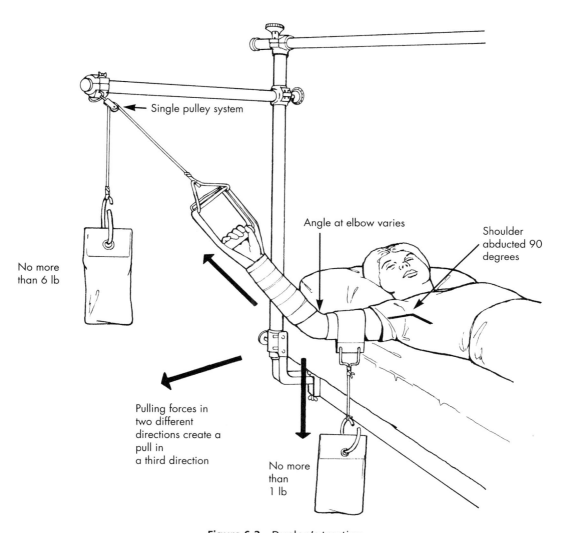

Single pulley system

Angle at elbow varies

Shoulder
abducted 90
degrees

No more
than 6 lb

Pulling forces in
two different
directions create a
pull in
a third direction

No more
than
1 lb

Figure 6-2 Dunlop's traction.

ing directly over the patient. Since the rope going through the pulleys extends in a straight line, the second pulley does not double the amount of pull, as in Russell's traction; rather the amount of pull remains the same as the amount of weight that is used.

Countertraction. Countertraction is usually adequately provided by the patient's own body weight. If additional countertraction is needed, 6-inch shock blocks can be placed under the legs of the bed on the same side of the traction force. There will be blocks under the wheels at the head and foot of the bed on the same side of the traction apparatus. Alternatively, you may place a folded blanket or sponge wedge between the mattress and the bed on the same side of the bed as the traction apparatus. This elevates the mattress slightly and provides the angle needed to accomplish countertraction.

Dunlop's Traction

Dunlop's traction is usually a temporary measure used in the treatment of transcondylar and supracondylar fractures of the humerus in children. These fractures present a serious problem, since perfect alignment of the bone fragments is needed to restore normal function at the elbow (Fig. 6-2).

Dunlop's traction incorporates a lateral pulling force to the elbow and a downward force on the distal portion of the upper arm. The pulling force is applied to the forearm laterally using skin traction. The downward force is applied by weights hanging from a sling positioned on the distal portion of the upper arm. This type of traction supports the arm in a position that allows for continuous pull in line with the humerus. Keeping the elbow flexed and applying traction at the lateral angle produce a traction pull in the longitudinal direction and stretch the biceps, which results in a molding force that helps bring the bone fragments into correct alignment. The line of pull may be altered by adjusting the weight or the angle at either the lateral arm traction or the sling.

Mechanical Components

Angles. The arm is held in a lateral position. The angle of the elbow varies because it must be adjusted by the physician as reduction occurs. The shoulder is abducted 90 degrees.

Weight. The weight applied by skin traction to the forearm should not exceed 6 pounds. That attached to the sling over the upper arm should not exceed 1 pound. This decreases the risk of neurovascular and skin integrity com-

promise. Be sure that the sling size is correct. It should not impair circulation to the elbow.

Pulleys. A single pulley system is attached to the skin traction. There are no pulleys needed for the second line of pull. This is accomplished by a sling applied over the upper arm to which a weight bag is attached.

Counteraction. Usually counteraction is adequately provided by the patient's own body weight. If additional countertraction is needed, 6-inch shock blocks can be placed under the legs of the bed on the same side as the traction force. There will be blocks under the wheels at the head and foot of the bed on the same side as the traction apparatus. Alternatively, you can place a folded blanket or sponge wedge between the mattress and the bed on the same side as the traction apparatus. This elevates the mattress slightly and provides the angle needed to accomplish countertraction.

Overhead 90-90 Traction

In overhead 90-90 traction the forearm is suspended over the upper chest of the patient. The humerus is perpendicular to the body and the elbow is flexed 90 degrees. The forearm rests in a supporting sling suspended from an overhead pulley (Fig. 6-3).

Overhead 90-90 traction is applied using a skeletal pin through the olecranon process of the ulna. The pin is usually of a small diameter (e.g., a Kirschner wire). The forearm is suspended in a sling to provide support and to help maintain position. It is not part of the traction pull.

Mechanical Components

Angles. The traction incorporates two 90-degree angles. One is made by the lines of the body and the humerus, the other by the lines

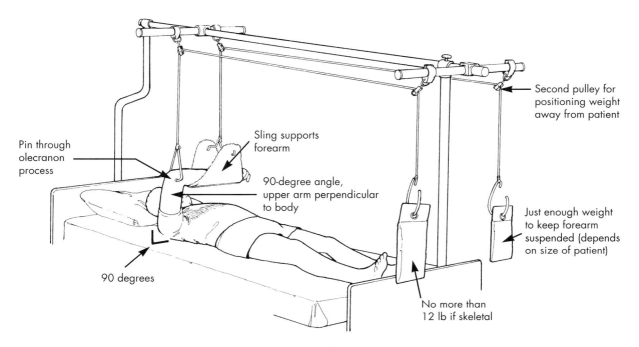

Pin through olecranon process

Sling supports forearm

90-degree angle, upper arm perpendicular to body

90 degrees

Second pulley for positioning weight away from patient

Just enough weight to keep forearm suspended (depends on size of patient)

No more than 12 lb if skeletal

Figure 6-3 Overhead 90-90 traction.

of the humerus and the forearm. The arm is perpendicular to the body, and the elbow is flexed at a 90-degree angle (Fig. 6-3).

Weight. For skeletal traction the weight should not exceed 12 pounds. The weight for suspension of the arm is attached to the sling. The amount of weight varies with the patient and is adjusted so the humerus is held perpendicular to the body. This helps maintain a 90-degree angle at the elbow.

Pulleys. There is a single pulley system applying force at the elbow. A second pulley system only holds the weights away from the patient and therefore does not bear on the amount of traction pull. The pulleys attached to the sling suspending the forearm are not incorporated into the traction pull but only suspend the upper arm to maintain the 90-degree angle.

Countertraction. Countertraction is accomplished by the weight of the patient's body.

Applying the Traction

Since traction application to the upper extremity can be either skin or skeletal, the nursing care for each patient must incorporate considerations for both types of traction.

For skin traction application, follow these directions:

- Assess the skin for potential breakdown. Skin traction should not be applied over an open wound, nor should it be applied to an extremity that has been abraded or lacerated or is infected.
- Assess for any allergies to adhesive tape or other materials that might be used in traction application.

- Assess the vascular and neurological status of the extremity before traction application.

If adhesive straps are used, the following points must be considered:

- Remove any hair from the extremity before application. Do this very carefully since even a minor irritation can cause problems if covered with adhesive straps for any length of time.
- Apply the straps to the skin from below the olecranon process of the ulna to just above the wrist.
- When the straps are in place, apply an elastic bandage. Wrap it snugly to prevent slipping but not so tight as to impair circulation. Part of the strap extends to the spreader bar, where the traction rope and weights will be attached.
- Apply a hand bar that is adjusted close enough to the patient's hand so the fingers will roll over the bar. This allows the hand to rest in a normal anatomical position and prevents it from flexing at the wrist and causing pressure on the radial nerve. Permanent disability, commonly known as "wrist drop," could result from radial nerve compression.
- Make sure that the spreader bar is wide enough to prevent the traction tapes from causing pressure on the lateral surfaces of the hand.
- For skeletal traction the pin inserted through the olecranon process of the ulna is small in diameter and therefore could cut through the bone if the amount of weight applied is too great. If the traction is used in children, the frequent movement of the child may cause the pin to slip.
- Make sure when applying 90-90 traction that the sling is the correct size. In over-

head 90-90 traction the sling should be large enough to incorporate the hand. If the sling is too small and does not adequately support the wrist and hand, pressure on the radial nerve could result, possibly causing wrist drop.

RELATED NURSING DIAGNOSES

Impaired Physical Mobility: Related to traction application and injury

Assessment	Rationale
Assess skin integrity on admission to hospital	May need to change treatment plan if open areas are present or skin is otherwise compromised
Assess alignment of body and upper extremity	For traction to be functioning properly, patient must be lying straight in bed
Check for proper application of traction apparatus	Decreases risk of skin breakdown, pain, and neurological deficit
Assess for straight line pull	Helps to minimize risk of malunion or nonunion
Assess neurological status	To identify compromise of radial nerve and therefore decrease risk of wrist drop
Assess ability to perform activities of daily living (ADLs)	May need assistance with daily hygiene and feeding

Interventions

1. Encourage the patient to do as much for himself or herself as possible. This helps the patient to move and increases self-esteem.

2. Encourage an exercise program to maintain strength, motion, and muscle tone in all muscles. These exercises can include

   a. Flexion and extension of the fingers: Instruct the patient to extend the fingers fully. Assess the neurovascular status of the hand and arm while this is being done. Evaluate each finger individually and document all symptoms (pain on movement, swelling, or change in temperature); report them immediately.

   b. Finger rolling: Instruct the patient to roll the fingers into a fist and hold tightly and then unroll and extend the fingers as far as possible.

   c. Flexion and extension of the wrist: Have the patient raise and lower the wrist in a waving motion. Use the wrist's full range of motion.

   d. Elbow exercises: In sidearm and Dunlop's traction the elbow must remain in a fixed position. In overhead 90-90 traction the physician may order exercises. Instruct the patient to flex and extend the elbow to the limits set by the physician. If needed, remove the sling to allow the prescribed movement. After exercising, make sure that the sling is appropriately placed so the wrist and hand have adequate support. Contact the occupational therapist or physical therapist for assistance in developing an exercise regimen for the patient.

   e. Instruct and help the patient perform full range-of-motion (ROM) exercises to the unaffected shoulder and elbow.

   f. Instruct the patient to perform range-of-motion exercises to all other joints. This will prevent venous stasis and maintain muscle tone when the patient is on prolonged bedrest. Recommended exercises are dorsiflexion and plantarflexion of the ankle, ankle circling, quadriceps setting of the thigh, and gluteal setting of the buttocks; also straight leg raising, knee flexion, and firmly pulling the heel toward the buttock. Exercise both lower extremities.

Impaired Skin Integrity: Related to immobility

Assessment	Rationale
Assess skin integrity on admission to hospital	To detect and document abrasions or bruising before traction is applied
Assess patient's complaints of discomfort	Pain or discomfort may indicate area of skin at risk before visible symptoms appear
Assess swelling of arm	Swelling increases risk of skin breakdown
Assess nutritional status and hydration	Patients who are malnourished or dehydrated are at increased risk of skin breakdown because of depleted protein stores and fluid deficiency
Assess mental status	Patients who are confused or agitated are more prone to skin breakdown with excessive motion; also prone to incontinence and noncompliance

Interventions

1. Observe the condition of the skin.

2. Keep the patient clean and dry.

3. Assess the extremity for swelling, especially around the elastic wrap.

4. Give skin care frequently. Administer skin care to the upper body as follows:

a. Instruct the patient to grasp the trapeze bar with the unaffected hand and bend the leg on the unaffected side.

b. While pulling up with the unaffected arm and pushing with the foot on the same side of the body, carefully roll the patient toward the affected side. Allow the patient to roll only enough for you to reach your hands under his back.

c. Visually inspect the skin of the back while the patient is in this position.

d. Change the bed linen while the patient is in this position. Place the linen lengthwise on the bed in a folded position and gently push the folds under the patient's shoulder. Do not pull the linen under the affected side but depress the mattress slightly and gently push the sheet under the patient. Make sure the linen is dry and wrinkle free.

e. Inspect the skin on the affected side; massage it by depressing the mattress.

f. Give skin care to the buttocks and coccyx by having the patient turn to one side while keeping the shoulders firmly against the bed.

g. Inspect the heels and massage them regularly since they are constantly pressed against the bed. Also observe the unaffected elbow for possible skin breakdown.

h. Observe the back of the head and ears. When the patient cannot use both shoulders to change position, the tendency is to press down on the back of the head for leverage. This can cause skin irritation and lead to breakdown.

5. Inspect the skin around the elastic wrap regularly. Since the arm is suspended, the potential for edema is minimal; therefore any edema that develops must be investigated. It might be caused by elastic wrap that is too tight

or by an impending compartment syndrome. Volkmann's contracture (ischemic muscle atrophy) is a serious complication caused by pressure on the nerves as they pass through the muscle and fascia. The result is a deformity consisting of a claw-shaped hand with flexed wrist and fingers and atrophy of the forearm.

6. Pin site care is also essential. Care for pin sites according to established procedure (hospital protocol or physician preference), observing carefully for slipping of the pin or evidence of the pin cutting through bone. The pin's diameter is small, and traction forces can cause the pin to slice into the bone.

Alteration in Comfort (Pain): Related to injury

Assessment	Rationale
Assess for signs and symptoms of pain or discomfort	May indicate ineffective treatment or improperly applied traction Indicates need to offer or administer analgesics May indicate possible complications (e.g., Volkmann's contracture)
Assess for increased pain on extension of fingers	May indicate compartment syndrome

Interventions

1. Administer analgesics as ordered, making sure to document the patient's response.

2. Teach the patient to use alternative methods of pain control to augment the use of medication. These include relaxation techniques and diversional activities such as reading, watching TV, or listening to the radio.

3. Reposition the patient or readjust the traction to help decrease the discomfort.

4. In children, investigate the integrity of the traction. If the child is old enough, ask him where it hurts. Medicate as ordered.

Self-Care Deficit: Inability to perform activities of daily living (ADLs) related to traction application and immobility

Assessment	Rationale
Assess for ability to perform ADLs	Patients in this type of traction have only one hand to use and will need assistance with all hygiene and other ADLs
Assess dietary needs	Patient may need assistance with meals as well as a nutritional consultation

Interventions

1. Assist the patient with self-care activities as needed.

2. Encourage the patient to do as much for himself as possible by placing essential equipment and articles within reach.

3. Monitor eating because swallowing in a supine position may be difficult.

4. Obtain a dietary consultation to determine which foods are easily swallowed and will provide the necessary nutrition.

High Risk for Peripheral Vascular Dysfunction: Related to traction application

Assessment	Rationale
Assess pulses distal to site of traction application and/or injury	Demonstrates presence or absence of arterial circulation distal to traction application or injury site
Assess capillary filling	Documents presence or absence of arterial return
Observe for swelling, warmth, and color of affected extremity as well as increased pain on passive motion of fingers	Complications such as compartment syndrome or Volkmann's contracture may be recognized and treated early
Assess for numbness, tingling, and loss of sensation	May indicate that elastic bandage is wrapped too tightly
Check for motor function	Inability to move fingers may indicate neurological damage

Interventions

1. Check for the presence and quality of pulses distal to (below) the injury or traction application site at least every 2 hours. To check capillary filling, use the blanching sign. Gently pinch the skin or nail bed of the affected extremity below the injury or site of traction application. The nail bed or skin should "blanch" or turn white. However, when the pressure of the pinch is eliminated, the area should return to its normal pink color. The rapidity with which this occurs demonstrates the presence or absence of capillary refill. If the skin does not return to its normal color within 2 to 4 seconds, suspect damage to the arterial circulation. Report and document these findings immediately. Poor capillary filling may indicate that the traction apparatus is applied too tightly or incorrectly or that there is an occult injury to the vascular system.

2. Compare the extremities for color, warmth, and swelling. Some residual swelling may exist from the original injury, but both extremities should be warm to the touch and their color should be about the same. If one

extremity is cool, has a whitish blue appearance, or has whitish blue nail beds, vascular integrity may be compromised. Report and document these findings immediately.

3. Ascertain if passive motion greatly increases pain. Gently move the fingers on the affected extremity. If the patient complains of extreme pain, beyond what would be expected, compartment syndrome may be present. (See Chapter 4.)

4. Ascertain if the patient is experiencing any pain, numbness, tingling, or loss of sensation in the affected extremity. Check for loss of sensation by gently touching the extremity with your hand or an open paper clip (being careful not to break the skin). Check for continued motor function by asking the patient to move the fingers of both extremities. Document any deficit and notify the physician immediately.

Impaired Gas Exchange: Related to immobility

Assessment	Rationale
Assess for breath sounds, respirations, and temperature	Prolonged bedrest in supine position may increase risk of respiratory problems

Interventions

1. Monitor vital signs, including temperature, pulse, respirations, and blood pressure.

2. Auscultate the lungs at least at every shift.

3. Encourage the patient to use incentive spirometry and to take deep breaths frequently.

4. Monitor eating to avoid the risk of aspiration.

5. Never leave a child in traction alone when eating.

6. Monitor the administration of medications that can cause respiratory depression.

Ineffective Coping: Related to immobility and hospitalization

Assessment	Rationale
Assess patient's ability and willingness to perform self-care activities; note any change in emotional status	Disinterest in personal hygiene may indicate depression
Evaluate patient's support systems	Support from family and friends is important in maintaining self-esteem and motivating patient to get well

Interventions

1. Develop a rapport with the patient.

2. Be aware of the normal grieving responses and allow the patient to express feelings openly.

3. Be aware of the resources available to the patient and be able to access these readily.

4. Encourage the family and friends to visit.

5. Allow the patient some time alone.

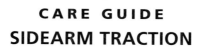

CARE GUIDE
SIDEARM TRACTION

The following information should be used in conjunction with the information found in the general traction management guide (Chapter 3).

MECHANICAL COMPONENTS

1. Weights . . . .
   a. Weight to forearm varies depending on size and weight of patient; this weight is not part of traction pull
   b. If traction pull is by skin method, amount of weight should not exceed 3 pounds; if pull is by skeletal method, amount of weight should not exceed 10 pounds.

2. Pulleys . . . .
   a. Two pulley systems; one is for suspension application, other for traction application
   b. Both are single-pulley systems; second apparatus is used to keep weights away from patient
   c. Pulleys are attached securely to bed frame

3. Ropes . . . .
   a. Freely movable and in pulley groove
   b. Knots secured with tape
   c. No kinks or fraying

4. Angles . . . .
   a. Pulling force to humerus is in lateral line; shoulder abducted 90 degrees from body and externally rotated; elbow flexed 90 degrees and held perpendicular to bed

5. Countertraction . . . .
   a. Provided by elevating side of bed; 6-inch shock blocks may be placed under wheels at head and foot of bed on same side as traction apparatus

b. Countertraction can also be provided by placing folded blanket or sponge wedge between mattress and bed frame on same side of bed as traction

6. Bed . . . .
a. Mattress is firm
b. Traction frame is securely attached, and all knobs are tight
c. Side rails cannot be used by patient on affected side but may be used on opposite side for leverage in moving

7. Trapeze . . . .
a. Patient may grasp it with unaffected hand and lift self for back care
b. Should be placed on traction frame at angle to allow unaffected elbow to be at 20 degrees (which is slightly anterior to level of shoulder)

PATIENT ALIGNMENT

1. Traction pull . . . .
a. Patient should be straight in bed
b. Frequent repositioning may be necessary to keep patient straight and maintain distance between spreader bar and pulleys

2. Provision of comfort when moving patient . .
a. Patient cannot be turned side to side; change position by having him or her pull on trapeze with unaffected arm and push up with feet

MAINTENANCE OF SKIN INTEGRITY

1. Check pressure points . . . .
a. Sacrum, heels, coccyx, spine, scapulae, back of head, affected shoulder and coccyx area; there is increased risk for patients with complicating problems (e.g., obesity, diabetes, paralysis, incontinence, or confusion)

2. Adjunct equipment to decrease risk
   of skin breakdown . . . .
   a. Use elbow protectors on unaffected side, heel protectors on both heels
   b. Pressure reduction mattress may be beneficial
   c. Do not use donut-type devices

EVALUATION OF AFFECTED EXTREMITY

1. Alteration in perfusion . . . .
   a. Check pulses distal to traction application site
   b. Check capillary filling
   c. Observe for warmth, color, and swelling
   d. Compare with unaffected extremity

2. Alteration in neurological status . . . .
   a. Check for numbness, tingling, pain, or pressure sensations
   b. Evaluate ability to move fingers

NURSING CARE

1. Alteration in gas exchange . . . .
   a. Instruct patient to take frequent deep breaths and to exhale forcibly
   b. Evaluate breath sounds regularly, especially on affected side

2. Alteration in nutritional status . . . .
   a. Offer foods that can be easily eaten such as finger foods
   b. Open all liquid containers and provide straws

3. Alteration in elimination . . . .
   a. Monitor bowel pattern carefully
   b. Offer bedpan from unaffected side, instructing patient to pull on trapeze with good hand and push up with feet
   c. Place call button within easy reach

4. Need for exercise . . . .
   a. Encourage exercise of unaffected arm, and lower extremities

b. Also encourage exercise of wrist and fingers of affected arm

5. Skin care related to application of traction

a. If traction and suspension applications are both by skin method, inspect extremity and skin over bony prominences

b. If application is by combination of skin and skeletal methods, follow procedure for pin site care

6. Ineffective coping . . . .

a. Explain all procedures

b. Give patient as much opportunity for independence as possible; keep necessary items within reach

c. All aspects of social implications need to be addressed

▼

CARE GUIDE
OVERHEAD 90-90

The following information should be used in conjunction with the information found in the general traction management guide (Chapter 3).

MECHANICAL COMPONENTS

1. Weights . . . .
   - a. Weight to forearm varies depending on size and weight of patient; this weight is applied to sling
   - b. Weight for traction pull is applied to arm:
     - (1) If pull is by skin method, amount of weight should not exceed 6 pounds
     - (2) If pull is by skeletal method, amount should not exceed 12 pounds

2. Pulleys . . . .
   - a. Two pulley systems; one is for suspension application, other for traction application
   - b. Both are single-pulley systems; second apparatus is used to keep weights away from patient
   - c. Pulleys are attached securely to bed frame

3. Ropes . . . .
   - a. Freely movable and in pulley groove
   - b. Knots secured with tape
   - c. No kinks or fraying

4. Angles . . . .
   - a. Upper arm is perpendicular to body, elbow flexed at 90 degree angle

5. Countertraction . . . .
   - a. Provided by weight of patient

6. Bed . . . .
   - a. Mattress is firm
   - b. Traction frame is securely attached, and all knobs are tight

	c. Side rails may be used on opposite side so patient can gain leverage for moving
7. Trapeze	a. May be used
	b. Should be attached at angle to allow unaffected elbow to be at 20 degrees to shoulder

PATIENT ALIGNMENT

1. Traction pull	a. Patient should be straight in bed
	b. Line of pull is vertical
2. Provision of comfort when moving patient . .	a. Patient cannot be turned side to side
	b. Change of position is achieved by having him or her pull on trapeze with unaffected arm and push up with feet

MAINTENANCE OF SKIN INTEGRITY

1. Check pressure points	a. Sacrum, heels, coccyx, spine, scapulae, and back of head
	b. Arm, wrist, and hand in sling must also be monitored
	c. Sling should be placed so it gives support to hand and does not cause pressure at wrist
3. Adjunct equipment to decrease skin breakdown	a. Use heel protectors on both heels, elbow protectors on unaffected side
	b. Pressure reduction mattress may be beneficial
	c. Do not use donut-type devices
	b. Soft padding material such as sheepskin may be used in the sling device

EVALUATION OF AFFECTED EXTREMITY

1. Alteration in perfusion	a. Check pulses distal to traction application site
	b. Check capillary filling

        c. Observe for warmth, color, and swelling

        d. Compare with unaffected extremity

2. Alteration in neurological status . . . .
        a. Check for numbness, tingling, pain, or pressure sensations

        b. Evaluate ability to move fingers

NURSING CARE

1. Alteration in gas exchange . . . .
        a. Instruct patient to take frequent deep breaths and to exhale forcefully

        b. Evaluate breath sounds regularly, especially on affected side (where secretions can pool)

2. Alteration in nutritional status . . . .
        a. Offer foods that can be easily eaten such as finger foods

        b. Open all liquid containers and provide straws

3. Alteration in elimination . . . .
        a. Monitor bowel pattern carefully

        b. Offer bedpan from unaffected side, instructing patient to pull on trapeze with good hand and push up with feet

        c. Place call button within easy reach

4. Need for exercise . . . .
        a. Encourage exercise of unaffected arm, lower extremities, wrist, and fingers of affected arm

5. Skin care related to application of traction . .
        a. Follow procedure for pin site care

        b. Sling supporting forearm may be moved for skin care and inspection

6. Ineffective coping . . . .
        a. Explain all procedures

        b. Give patient as much opportunity for independence as possible; keep necessary items within reach

        c. All aspects of social implications need to be addressed

▼

CARE GUIDE
DUNLOP'S TRACTION

The following information should be used in conjunction with the information found in the general traction management guide (Chapter 3).

MECHANICAL COMPONENTS

1. Weights . . . .
   a. Amount of weight applied by skin traction to forearm should not exceed 6 pounds, and weight attached to sling over upper arm should not exceed 1 pound
   b. Since this type of traction is used mainly in children, specific orders on amount of weight should be written by physician

2. Pulleys . . . .
   a. Single-pulley system is attached to traction application
   b. Second traction force is applied by means of sling over upper arm

3. Ropes . . . .
   a. Freely movable and in pulley groove
   b. Knots secured with tape
   c. No kinks or fraying

4. Angles . . . .
   a. Arm is held in lateral position; angle of elbow is 45 degrees, but may be adjusted by physician to facilitate reduction of fracture
   b. Shoulder is abducted 90 degrees

5. Countertraction . . . .
   a. Provided by elevating side of bed on same side as traction apparatus
   b. Shock blocks may be placed under wheels of one side of bed at the head and foot

6. Bed . . . .
  a. Mattress is firm
  b. Traction frame is securely attached, and all knobs are tight
  c. Side rails cannot be used by patient on affected side but may be used on opposite side for leverage in moving

7. Trapeze . . . .
  a. Patient may grasp it and lift self
  b. Should be placed on traction frame at angle to allow unaffected elbow to be at 20 degrees (which is slightly anterior to level of shoulder)

PATIENT ALIGNMENT

1. Traction pull . . . .
  a. Patient should be straight in bed
  b. Line of pull varies as angle of traction is adjusted by physician

2. Provision of comfort when moving patient
  a. Patient cannot be turned side to side; change of position is achieved by having him or her pull on trapeze with unaffected arm and push up with feet
  b. If traction frame is attached to movable part of bed frame, head of bed may be elevated for comfort and for eating
  c. Since countertraction is accomplished by elevating side of bed, patient may slide to that side; sheet restraint may be used to help keep this from happening

MAINTENANCE OF SKIN INTEGRITY

1. Check pressure points . . . .
  a. Sacrum, heels, coccyx, spine, scapulae, back of head, affected shoulder
  b. Sling should be placed so as not to cause pressure in antecubital space

2. Adjunct equipment to decrease risk
   of skin breakdown . . . . a. Use heel protectors on both heels, elbow protectors on unaffected side
   b. Pressure reduction mattress may be used
   c. Do not use donut-type devices
   d. Soft padding material such as sheepskin may be used in sling

EVALUATION OF AFFECTED EXTREMITY

1. Alteration in perfusion . . . . a. Instruct patient to take frequent deep breaths and to exhale forcibly
   b. Evaluate breath sounds regularly, especially on affected side (where secretions can pool)

2. Alteration in neurological status . . . . a. Check pulses distal to traction application site
   b. Check capillary filling
   c. Observe for warmth, color, and swelling
   d. Compare with unaffected extremity

2. Alteration in nutritional status . . . . a. Offer foods that can be easily eaten such as finger foods
   b. Open all liquid containers and provide straws

3. Alteration in elimination . . . . a. Monitor bowel pattern carefully
   b. Offer bedpan from unaffected side, instructing patient to pull on trapeze with unaffected hand and push up with feet
   c. Place call button within easy reach

4. Need for exercise . . . . a. Encourage exercise of unaffected arm, and lower extremities
   b. Also encourage exercise of wrist and fingers of affected arm

5. Skin care related to application of traction

    a. Check skin traction for tightness and to ensure that it has not slipped and is not causing pressure at wrist

    b. Sling hanging over upper arm may be moved for skin care and inspection only with specific instructions from physician

6. Ineffective coping . . . .

    a. Explain all procedures

    b. Give patient as much opportunity for independence as possible; keep necessary items within reach

    c. Since this is usually temporary traction, planning for ongoing care should begin immediately

    d. Involvement of parents or other caregivers for pediatric patient is essential

7 Traction to the Spine

When the spine becomes diseased or is injured, the treatment of choice may be traction. Several modalities can be used depending on the severity and location of the disease or injury.

Cervical Traction

Circumferential head halter traction (Fig. 7-1) applies skin traction to the cervical spine using a halter that encircles the head (back of the skull and under the chin). It is used, often intermittently, in the treatment of cervical sprains and strains, ruptured cervical discs, nerve impingement from degenerative diseases (arthritis), and torticollis. It can be used as a temporary method of immobilization while minor cervical vertebral fractures or subluxations are being ruled out. It may also be used to immobilize the cervical spine or gently pull the cervical vertebrae apart, relieving pressure on the spinal nerves.

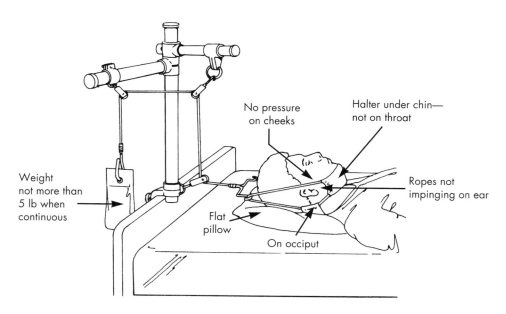

No pressure on cheeks

Halter under chin— not on throat

Weight not more than 5 lb when continuous

Ropes not impinging on ear

Flat pillow

On occiput

Figure 7-1 Circumferential head halter traction.

Mechanical Components

Angles. The traction pull is delivered in a straight line from the halter off the end of the bed. A straight line is maintained to avoid angulation of the cervical spine.

Weight. To prevent skin breakdown or discomfort in the jaw, the weight used for continuous halter traction rarely exceeds 5 pounds. In intermittent use (for nerve impingement, etc.) the weight may be as great as 10 to 15 pounds for a period of 15 to 20 minutes.

Pulleys. The type of equipment used to apply this traction varies by hospital. Some devices attach to the head of the bed with an adjustable single pulley. This allows the head of the bed to be raised and lowered while maintaining the straight line pull of the traction. The pulley can be raised or lowered separately to alter the direction of the traction force to fit individual needs.

Countertraction. If the patient must remain flat in bed, countertraction may be provided by elevating the head of the bed with 6-inch blocks or a reverse Trendelenburg. To apply the traction apparatus, you may have to place the patient with his head at the foot of the bed, which may be elevated. Countertraction may also be provided by the patient's body weight.

Applying the Head Halter

1. Center the halter evenly on the chin so there is no pressure on the throat. The pull of the traction should be on the occipital area. Ensure that the spreader bar is wide enough to avoid pressure on the sides of the head and allow the ears to remain free. After applying the halter properly, attach the spreader bar by looping the ropes of the halter around the bar, securing them at the distal grooves (Fig. 7-1).

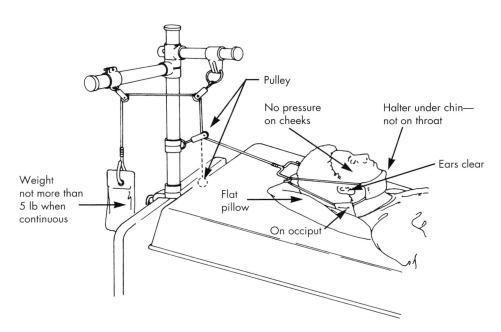

Figure 7-2 Head halter traction using an adjustable pulley.

Then tie a rope to the spreader bar, thread it through the pulley(ies), and attach it to the weight. Apply the weight slowly and cautiously, being careful not to drop the weights or jar the patient.

2. When applying cervical circumferential traction to males, discuss the issue of beard growth with the patient; this may be a source of discomfort during treatment. Encourage the patient to remain clean shaven.

3. Position the patient straight in the center of the bed where the spreader bar does not reach the pulley. Patients should rest on their back with their shoulders level to maintain the desired line of pull. You may place a small pillow or bath blanket under the head and flex the knees slightly either by elevating the knee gatch or by placing a pillow under them.

4. When using an adjustable pulley apparatus, elevate the head of the bed while maintaining the line of pull. Move the adjustable pulley to maintain the prescribed line of pull (Fig. 7-2).

5. When a bed with an adjustable pulley is not available or the patient must remain flat on the bed in cervical traction, you may need to change the patient's position so the head is at the foot of the bed. Keep the mattress level with the foot of the bed so the traction pull remains in a straight line. You may need a second mattress to maintain the desired level.

RELATED NURSING DIAGNOSES

Impaired Physical Mobility: Related to prolonged bedrest

Assessment	Rationale
Assess skin integrity on admission to hospital	May need to change treatment plan if open areas are present or if skin is otherwise compromised

Assessment	Rationale
Assess alignment of patient's body	To function properly, patient must lie straight in bed
Check for proper application of halter	Decreases risk of skin breakdown and possible jaw pain
Assess for straight line of pull	Minimizes risk of angulating cervical vertebrae
Assess neurological status	Patients treated with cervical traction have injuries or conditions that predispose to neurological deficits
Assess ability to perform ADLs	Needed to determine level of assistance required (if traction is intermient, patient may be able to perform most functions on his own)

Interventions

1. Turn and reposition the patient every 2 hours if allowed.

2. Teach the patient how to get up without increasing discomfort or risking further injury if the traction is ordered intermittently and the patient is allowed out of bed. To do this:

    a. Remove the halter.

    b. Instruct the patient to log-roll onto side and push the upper body up in one, smooth, straight motion while simultaneously allowing the legs to move over the side of the bed, keeping the back and neck straight.

    c. Stand at the side of the bed toward which the patient will be getting up so you will be in front of the patient when he is sitting on the edge of the bed.

3. Instruct the patient not to lift with the head (as in a sit-up) because this causes undue strain on the neck.

4. Avoid using a trapeze for cervical traction patients because it may interfere with the line of pull.

5. Encourage the patient to do as much for himself as possible to encourage movement and increase self-esteem.

6. Encourage participation in an exercise program to help maintain motion, strength, and muscle tone.

Potential for Impaired Skin Integrity:
Related to traction application

Assessment	Rationale
Assess skin integrity on admission to hospital	May need to change treatment plan if open areas are present or if skin is otherwise compromised
Assess patient's complaints of discomfort	Discomfort may indicate area of concern not evident on initial examination
Assess for areas of swelling	Pressure from halter on a swollen head, neck, or jaw can cause skin breakdown
Assess nutritional status	A malnourished (depleted protein stores) or dehydrated patient is at increased risk of skin breakdown
Assess mental status	A confused or agitated patient is prone to skin breakdown because of excessive movement; also prone to incontinence and noncompliance
Assess all skin that comes in contact with halter	Decreases risk of skin breakdown

Assessment	Rationale
Inspect skin at least every 2 to 3 hours	Allows potential skin problems to be recognized and treated immediately
Inspect bed linens and change as needed	Changing soiled linen in timely manner decreases risk of skin breakdown

Interventions

1. Alleviate excessive pressure on the skin by using special mattress or sheepskin, positioning the patient with pillows, applying special protectors (heel and elbow) or using a therapeutic bed.

2. Do not seat the patient on a rubber ring or doughnut; these appliances restrict circulation to the coccyx, which increases the risk of skin breakdown.

3. Encourage the patient to eat a diet that provides adequate protein and calories.

4. Encourage adequate fluid intake to prevent dehydration. The suggested intake for a patient with no medical restrictions is approximately 2600 ml over 24 hours.

5. Encourage the patient to do as much as possible for himself or herself.

6. Encourage participation in an exercise program to maintain motion, strength, and muscle tone.

7. Reinforce the patient's orientation to time, place, and self if needed. Have family members bring in familiar objects or pictures. Keep a small light on at night.

Applying Circumferential Cervical Traction

1. Carefully examine the areas of skin that will contact the halter, including the chin, jaw, ears, cheeks, and occipital region.

2. Make sure that there is no pressure on the throat. The pull should be on the occipital area.

3. After traction has been applied, check these areas every 2 to 3 hours for redness, blisters, or breakdown.

4. Make sure that the ropes of the halter fit loosely over the cheeks to avoid cutting into the skin and to prevent facial nerve damage.

5. Teach the patient to remove and reapply the halter if allowed.

6. Explain how to establish that the traction is effective by evaluating the placement of the ropes, pulleys, and spreader bar and by observing the decrease in symptoms.

7. Establish a schedule for removal and reapplication of the traction if the patient is unable to do this.

8. Change the halter as needed.

9. Sprinkle talcum powder or cornstarch on the area covered by the halter (especially the chin area) to decrease moisture and irritation.

Pain: Related to injury or prolonged bedrest

Assessment	Rationale
Assess for signs and symptoms of pain or discomfort	May indicate inappropriate treatment or improperly applied traction
	Indicates need to offer or administer analgesics
	May indicate complication
Assess for pain in jaw	May indicate temporomandibular joint (TMJ) problem or inappropriate application of head halter
Assess for facial pain	May indicate facial nerve problem

Interventions

1. Establish a routine for removal and reapplication of the head halter.

2. If permitted, allow for time out of traction to decrease pressure on the nerves and joints.

3. Assess for skin irritation or breakdown, distended bladder, or excessive swelling of the limbs.

4. Position the patient on either side, if able, to minimize discomfort and decrease the risk of skin breakdown. If allowed, the patient may be supported with pillows while on his side for short periods.

5. Apply a cervical collar, if ordered, while the patient is up and out of bed. This helps to support the head and neck and decreases discomfort. Fit the collar properly. (See the manufacturer's instructions for measurement and application.)

6. Encourage use of a mouthguard, similar to the ones used by athletes, to reduce discomfort caused by pressure on the TMJ. Pain from pressure on the TMJ may be referred to the middle ear or throat and interfere with chewing.

7. Check the amount of weight. Too much may cause headaches because of overpull or improper pull on the cervical musculature.

8. Administer analgesics as ordered.

9. Report any pain in the traction area to the physician immediately, especially if not responsive to medication.

Self-Care Deficits: Related to position and neurological status. (Inability to perform activities of daily living [ADLs] may be due to weakness of the upper extremities.)

Assessment	Rationale
Assess for ability to perform ADLs	Patient may need assistance with hygiene, feeding, and toileting

Assessment	Rationale
Assess patient's ability to chew and swallow	May need to modify diet to decrease risk of choking, may also indicate trigeminal nerve irritation

Interventions

1. Encourage the patient to perform as many self-care activities as possible, especially if the traction can be removed and the patient is allowed out of bed.

2. Instruct the patient how to get out of bed. (See p. 68.)

3. Modify the diet as necessary, adding soft foods and foods that require minimal chewing.

4. Add dietary supplements to ensure that the patient obtains adequate nutritional support.

5. Monitor eating and drinking, especially if choking or vomiting is possible.

6. Educate all personnel caring for the patient as to the proper method for removing the halter in case of an emergency, such as vomiting.

7. Keep the halter off for a short time after meals (if possible) to allow the patient to begin digestion. This helps decrease the risk of regurgitation.

High Risk for Peripheral Vascular Dysfunction

Assessment	Rationale
Assess neurological status	May indicate extension of cervical injury or disease
Assess for Radial pulses Pedal pulses Temperature of skin Triceps reflex Biceps reflex Knee reflex	Any deficit could indicate extension of injury or improper application of traction

Assessment	Rationale
Ankle reflex Motion of all four extremities Sensation of all four extremities	
Assess for facial pain, loss of sensation, or motor weakness	May indicate irritation or pressure on trigeminal or facial nerves (**trigeminal:** pain or loss of sensation in face, forehead, temple, and eye; deviation of jaw toward the paralyzed side, and difficulty chewing; **facial:** paralysis of all muscles on one side of face, inability to wrinkle forehead, close eye, or whistle, deviation of mouth to unaffected side)

Interventions

1. Check the vascular system:
   a. Note the presence and quality of pulses in all four extremities
   b. Assess capillary refill time of the fingers and toes by using the blanching sign, which evaluates arterial return. Gently pinch the skin or nail bed of any of the extremities. The nail bed should "blanch" or turn white; then, as soon as the pressure of the pinch is released, the area should return to its normal pink color. The rapidity with which this occurs demonstrates the presence or absence of capillary refill.
   If the skin does not return to its normal color within 2 to 4 seconds, compromise of the vascular system must to be ruled out. Document and report these findings to the physician immediately.

2. Evaluate the neurological status:
   a. Ask the patient if he or she is experiencing pain, numbness, tingling, or loss of sensation in any extremity. Check for sensation by gently touching the extremity with an open paper clip, being careful not to break the skin. Assessing numbness and tingling of a patient in head halter traction is important because pressure on the spinal cord from degenerative diseases increases over time. If the patient experiences a change or increase in symptoms, another form of treatment may be needed.
   b. Check for continued motor function by asking the patient to move his fingers, toes, arms, and legs.
   c. If any deficit is noted, document and report it to the physician immediately.
3. Use of the head halter may place undue pressure on the trigeminal and/or facial nerves. If the patient experiences pain or loss of sensation in the face, forehead, temple, or eye and complains of difficulty chewing, with a demonstrated deviation of the jaw toward one side, the trigeminal nerve may be compromised. If the patient is unable to move any muscles on one side of the face, to wrinkle the forehead, or to close the eye, or if there is deviation of the mouth toward one side, the facial nerve may be involved. These should be documented and reported to the physician immediately. You may need to remove the traction, sandbag the head, or apply a cervical collar. However, these should be done only with a physician's order.

Alteration in Gas Exchange: Related to traction apparatus and position

Assessment	Rationale
Assess respiratory status; auscultate lungs for Rales Rhonchi Wheezing Decreased breath sounds	May indicate hypostatic pneumonia
Assess vital signs: Temperature Pulse Respirations	Needed to recognize early signs of hypostatic pneumonia
Assess for proper application of halter	Avoid halter pressure on trachea or jaw

Interventions

1. Ensure that the head halter is applied appropriately and does not press on any structures that might interfere with breathing.

2. Make sure that all personnel involved with care of the patient can quickly remove the halter apparatus if choking or respiratory difficulty occurs.

3. Have sandbags or a soft collar readily available.

4. Keep oxygen and suction at the bedside for immediate use.

5. Monitor the patient during meals, and modify the diet if necessary to include softer foods that decrease chewing time and the risk of choking.

Ineffective Coping: Related to injury, disease, and fear of permanent paralysis

Assessment	Rationale
Assess patient's ability to perform self-care activities; also note any changes in emotional response	Disinterest in personal hygiene may indicate depression

Assessment	Rationale
Assess patient's support systems	Support from family and friends helps to maintain self-esteem and motivate patient to get well; also helps to determine appropriate resources to contact if needed
Assess patient's level of anxiety	Cervical injury or disease is frightening and may focus patient's thoughts on threat of permanent paralysis

Interventions

1. Adequately explain all procedures to both the patient and the family or significant other.

2. Allow the patient to do as much for himself or herself as possible.

3. Be aware that the patient may not be able to see the surroundings; stand in plain view well within the patient's line of vision.

4. Place call bells and other necessary equipment within easy reach.

5. Provide prism glasses to facilitate reading or watching television if the patient cannot be up or have the head of the bed elevated.

6. Determine the patient's support systems.

7. Access appropriate resources when needed: social worker, psychologist or psychiatrist, chaplain.

8. Develop a rapport with the patient and allow time for the patient to talk without interruption or the feeling of being judged.

9. Arrange for the patient to spend some time without distraction (quiet time).

Skeletal Cervical Traction

Skeletal traction to the cervical spine works by direct fixation to the skull. Cervical tongs (Gardner-Wells, Crutchfield, Vinke) or a halo vest apparatus is attached to the skull through predrilled holes into the outer layer of the cranium. The halo can be used for skeletal traction, or it may be attached to a vest by metal bars to provide rigid fixation of the spine. Although technically not traction, this mechanism holds the spine in alignment after the fracture has been reduced (Figs. 7-3 and 7-4). For cervical traction, first a local anesthetic is instilled; then the holes are made with a special drill. As with skeletal traction of the upper and lower extremities, this type of cervical traction is always continuous.

Skeletal traction to the spine is used for fractures or dislocations of the cervical vertebrae and high thoracic fractures where the spine is unstable and injury to the spinal cord is possible. It is used to reduce cervical subluxations and in scoliosis treatment. The halo vest is often used for immobilizing a neurologically intact patient with an unstable fracture or dislocation. It may be employed to maintain stability during surgery and, along with the torso vest, after surgery to facilitate mobility. Halo jackets are not recommended for patients with

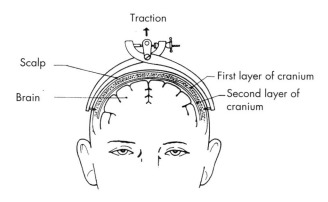

Figure 7-3   Cervical tongs.

Emergency Removal of Chest Plate

Patient lies supine in bed.

Unscrew bolt at each end of
bar on front of chest plate.

Move bars laterally.

Loosen buckle on each
shoulder.

Loosen buckle on each
side at bottom of vest.

Slide vest off.

Keep wrench taped to chest
plate *at all times*.

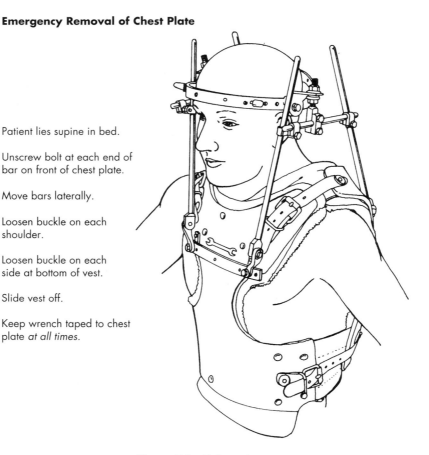

Figure 7-4   Halo vest.

respiratory insufficiency because they constrict
the chest area.

The halo is a metal ring attached to the patient's head with two anterior and two posterior pins. The pins are placed in the operating
room under sterile conditions. The halo is attached to the pins and then to a vest by four
lightweight metal bars. The vest is usually made
of plastic with a sheepskin lining. Sometimes
the vest can be removed for skin care and
changing of the lining. All personnel caring for
the patient in a halo vest should know how to

remove the vest quickly in case of an emergency, such as cardiac arrest. The proper
equipment (i.e., wrench) should be available
for ready removal; one excellent recommenda-
tion is to tape it directly to the front of the vest.

Sometimes the vest is made of plaster of
Paris. The four lightweight bars are incorporated into the plaster at the time of application.

Mechanical Components

Pulleys. Cervical traction uses a single pulley
system. Depending on the type of fracture, the

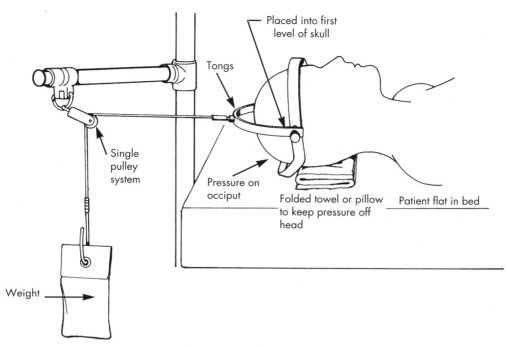

Figure 7-5 Halo traction.

head of the bed may be gatched to hyperextend the neck and thereby facilitate reduction.

Angles. The line of pull along the cervical vertebrae is adjusted to align the fragments and protect the spinal cord. The direction of pull can be altered by changing the degree of extension or flexion of the neck (Fig. 7-5).

Weights. Weights vary according to the condition of the patient and the type of traction. A standard method is to use a 10-pound base and add 5 pounds for each vertebrae from C-3 to the level of the fracture. Not uncommonly 35 pounds of weight may be used to reduce a fracture at the C-7 level (Fig. 7-5). Frequent x-rays are taken to monitor the progress of the reduction. Once the fracture is reduced, the physician may order a decrease in weight. If the patient is elderly or has severe degenerative

changes, less weight may be needed. The physician must carefully monitor the patient's progress with x-ray control.

Countertraction. Countertraction is provided by the patient's body weight. The bed is placed in a reverse Trendelenburg position if the amount of weight needed for reduction of the fracture exceeds 15 to 20 pounds. Countertraction may also be provided by elevating the head of the bed approximately 6 inches. If a nonelectric bed is used, the patient's head is placed at the foot of the bed. The footboard of the bed is usually lower than the headboard and can accommodate the traction assembly and maintain the traction in a straight line. A turning frame (e.g., Stryker frame) or other type of therapeutic bed may be used if the patient cannot be safely turned in a conventional bed.

The patient is positioned in the center of the bed, situated so the tongs or halo do not rest against the pulley. The patient should lie on his back with the shoulders level.

Use of a trapeze is unsafe for a patient in skeletal cervical traction. Any change in the alignment resulting from extending or flexing the neck can cause serious injury to the spinal cord. The degree of extension or flexion of the neck may be adjusted only by the physician.

RELATED NURSING DIAGNOSES

Impaired Physical Mobility: Related to bedrest and injury

Assessment	Rationale
Assess skin integrity on admission to hospital	May need to change treatment plan if open areas are present or if skin is otherwise compromised
Assess alignment of body	For traction to function properly, patient must be lying straight in bed
Inspect pin sites	If there is redness, drainage, or pin migration, or if pins become infected or loose, treatment may need to be changed
Assess for straight line of pull	Minimizes risk of angulation of cervical vertebrae
Assess patient's ability to be turned	As soon as possible, must institute a turning schedule to maintain skin integrity without compromising neurological status

Assessment	Rationale
Assess neurological status	Patients treated by cervical traction have injuries or conditions that can predispose to neurological deficits
Assess ability to perform ADLs	Patients treated by skeletal cervical traction are usually flat in bed and may be unable to perform even basic hygiene functions

Interventions

1. Institute an exercise program that includes dorsiflexion and plantarflexion of the ankles, ankle circling, quadriceps setting, and flexing of the hips and knees if possible.

2. Include upper extremity range-of-motion (ROM) exercises in the program.

3. Make sure that all exercises are individualized for the patient and a doctor's order is on the chart for any exercise program.

4. Provide for passive ROM exercises if neurological deficit is present.

5. Arrange for functional bracing of the extremities once the degree of paralysis has been established.

6. Increase activity as tolerated once the patient's condition is stabilized.

7. Consult physical therapy and occupational therapy to provide appropriate exercises and bracing.

8. Make sure that the physician's **order for turning** the patient is written on the record. If the patient is in a conventional bed, follow this protocol:

a. Explain to the patient exactly what will be done.

b. Use at least two people.

c. Position one person to support and guide the head and neck and the other to turn the patient's body simultaneously.

d. Log-roll the patient to a position of comfort, usually 30 to 45 degrees on either side.

e. If the patient can remain on the side for short periods, position and support the body and head with pillows.

f. Maintain the traction in a straight line.

Alteration in Skin Integrity: Related to bedrest and neurological deficit

Assessment	Rationale
Assess skin integrity on admission to hospital	May need to change treatment plan if open areas are present or if skin integrity is otherwise compromised
Assess patient's complaints of discomfort	May indicate area of concern not evident on initial examination; or may signify return of neurological function
Assess nutritional status and hydration	Malnourished (depleted protein stores) or dehydrated patient is at increased risk of skin breakdown
Assess pin sites	To prevent pin site infection
Assess occiput	To prevent skin breakdown

Assessment	Rationale
Assess mental status	Confused or agitated patient more prone to skin breakdown resulting from excessive movement, incontinence, or noncompliance
Inspect skin at least every 2 to 3 hours	Potential skin problems may be recognized and treated immediately
Inspect bed linen and change as needed	Changing soiled linen in timely manner decreases risk of skin breakdown

Interventions

1. Assess all bony prominences, including the occiput. This area is vulnerable to skin breakdown, especially if the patient cannot be turned.

2. Examine the occiput at least every 2 to 3 hours for redness, blistering, or open areas.

3. Place a thin piece of foam rubber under the head for cushioning, if possible.

4. Provide skin care by depressing the mattress enough to extend a hand under the patient to massage the skin. This is less than satisfactory and should be used only until the exact extent of the injury is determined.

5. Consult with the physician about placing the patient in a therapeutic bed. (See Chapter 10.)

6. Massage the skin of the back, heels, and elbows with a lubricant to keep the skin supple.

7. Massage the lubricant completely into the skin to decrease the chance of moisture buildup, especially in the coccygeal area.

8. Alleviate pressure on bony prominences by using a special mattress, overlay, or therapeutic bed.

9. Avoid using a donut or rubber ring; these devices restrict the circulation to the coccyx and increase the risk of skin breakdown.

10. Inspect the skin under the halo vest if the patient is being treated in this apparatus. Areas of concern are the axillae and the torso.

11. Change the sheepskin padding of the halo vest if it becomes soiled; follow the manufacturer's recommendations.

12. Provide routine cast care if the jacket is made of plaster of Paris.

13. Keep the cast dry and clean.

14. Petal the edges of the cast with tape to prevent skin irritation and to keep flakes of plaster from falling under the cast.

15. Inspect the skin for any signs of redness, blistering, or broken areas.

16. Be aware that the patient with neurological deficits may not be able to communicate any feelings of discomfort or pain.

Pain: Related to injury

Assessment	Rationale
Assess for signs and symptoms of discomfort	May indicate inappropriate treatment or improperly applied traction
	Indicates need to offer or administer analgesics
	May indicate complications (e.g., DVT)
Assess neurological status	Patient may not be able to communicate pain or discomfort
Assess for bladder distention and swelling of extremities	Patient may not be able to communicate pain or discomfort

Interventions

1. Evaluate the patient for situations in which pain might be a major symptom (e.g., DVT, urinary retention, or skin breakdown).

2. Establish a turning schedule.

3. Monitor intake and output.

4. Obtain an order for an indwelling catheter or to begin intermittent catheterization if needed.

5. Monitor any swelling of the extremities.

6. Administer analgesics as ordered.

7. Be aware that a head injury may accompany a cervical injury and narcotics may be contraindicated.

8. Teach the patient alternative methods of pain control such as relaxation techniques or guided imagery.

9. Encourage diversional activities as tolerated.

Self-Care Deficit: Related to position and neurological status

Assessment	Rationale
Assess for ability to perform ADLs	Need to determine level of activity; specifically, does patient require help with feeding, bathing, or toileting?

Interventions

1. Devise a turning schedule.

2. Change the patient's position as often as every 2 hours.

3. Maintain the extremities in functional positions.

4. Consult occupational therapy for functional bracing.

5. Provide assistance with all ADLs as needed.

6. Maintain privacy and dignity when assisting with toileting.

7. Institute a bowel- and bladder-retraining program as soon as possible (if necessary).

8. Monitor the patient while feeding to prevent choking and aspiration.

9. Make sure that oxygen and suction are available for use in an emergency.

10. Encourage the patient to do as much self-care as possible. This fosters movement, helps maintain a level of independence, and increases self-esteem.

11. Devise an exercise program with the help of physical therapy personnel.

Alteration in Gas Exchange: Related to injury

Assessment	Rationale
Assess respiratory status	Depending on level of injury, patient may require mechanical ventilation
Auscultate lungs	Watch for symptoms of respiratory distress or pneumonia

Interventions

1. Monitor for signs and symptoms of hypostatic pneumonia (i.e., increased respiratory rate, dyspnea, cyanosis, elevated temperature, lung congestion, pleuritic chest pain, lethargy).

2. Turn the patient at least every 2 hours to facilitate movement of secretions.

3. Auscultate for breath sounds at least every 2 hours initially.

4. Maintain a patent airway.

5. Notify the physician immediately if the patient develops acute respiratory distress. Mechanical ventilation via an endotracheal tube or tracheostomy may be needed.

6. Be aware that hyperextension of the patient's neck to insert the endotracheal tube may be impossible.

7. Use caution when administering drugs that decrease the rate and depth of lung expansion (i.e., narcotics for analgesia).

8. Encourage deep breathing and incentive spirometry use as tolerated.

Ineffective Coping: Related to actual or threatened paralysis

Assessment	Rationale
Assess patient's ability to perform self-care activities; note any changes in emotional responses	Disinterest in personal hygiene may indicate depression
Evaluate patient's support system	Support from family and friends helps maintain self-esteem and motivate patient to get well
Assess patient's level of anxiety	Cervical injury is frightening and may focus patient's thoughts on threat of permanent paralysis
Assess for appropriate resource referrals	Patient and family may need support from resources such as psychology, social services, or pastoral counseling

Interventions

1. Provide adequate explanations for all procedures to both the patient and the family or significant other.

2. Allow the patient to do as much self-care as possible.

3. Stand in the patient's line of vision as needed since the patient may be unable to see his surroundings secondary to being flat and unable to move.

4. Place the call bell and other necessary equipment within easy reach of the patient.

5. Teach the patient to use the call system, especially if it is specifically adapted for use by neurologically impaired patients.

6. Evaluate (with the physician and other disciplines) the permanency of the patient's deficit. Life-style changes for patient, family, and significant other may be drastic and permanent.

7. Access appropriate resources as needed (e.g., psychological services, social services, or pastoral services).

8. Encourage family and friends to visit.

9. Allow the patient to speak freely without fear of being judged.

10. Allow the patient some time alone.

11. Encourage mobilization if appropriate.

12. Be aware that the patient may have difficulty with altered body image and may withdraw, refusing to participate in activities.

13. Develop a rapport with the patient and family or significant other.

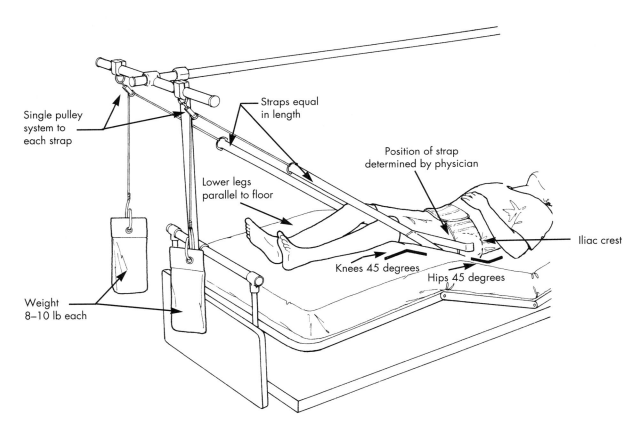

Figure 7-6 Circumferential skin traction to the lumbar spine (pelvic traction).

Pelvic Traction: Circumferential Skin Traction to the Lumbar Spine

Pelvic traction is applied to the lumbar spine by means of a pelvic belt placed just above and around the iliac crests. It is used to manage acute and chronic low back pain, a herniated lumbar disc, and degenerative arthritis of the lumbar spine. The traction is applied with the patient in the Williams position, with the hips and knees both flexed approximately 45 degrees. The lower legs are kept parallel to the floor, and the head of the bed is elevated 20 to 30 degrees. (See Figure 7-6.)

Mechanical Components

Angles. The pulling force is aligned with the axis of the femur. The patient is in the Williams position. The belt is applied according to the direction of the pull. If it is applied with the straps parallel to the thigh, the pull will be directed downward; if applied with the straps placed posteriorly, the pelvis will be pulled into a "tucked-in" position. The physician determines the placement of the straps.

Weights. Because the belt is applied directly to the skin, the amount of weight should rarely exceed 8 to 10 pounds to each strap. This will decrease the risk of skin irritation or breakdown.

Pulleys. Pelvic traction utilizes two single-pulley systems. Each strap has its own pulley.

Countertraction. Countertraction is provided by the weight of the patient in bed.

Applying the Belt

The pelvic belt encircles the pelvis over the iliac crest and is fastened with Velcro straps or buckles. It is applied directly to the skin. Since belts come in various sizes, check the manufacturer's specifications for measuring and applying the belt.

After the belt is applied, attach the straps at the bottom edge of the belt extending to the pulleys and weights at the foot of the bed. Adjust the strap lengths so there are equal lengths to both sides for equal pull. To avoid friction, which decreases the efficiency of traction, the straps must clear the bed as they extend to the pulleys.

The Williams position must be maintained to ensure that the therapeutic value of this form of treatment is obtained. Instruct the patient not to lie flat with the hips and knees extended because this causes hyperextension of the lumbar spine and increases pain.

The traction may be uncomfortable if applied for long periods; therefore intermittent application is usually ordered. When reapplied, the straps must be in the prescribed place.

The Pelvic Sling

The pelvic sling is used to stabilize and immobilize fractures of the pelvis and to treat separation of the anterior pelvic ring. It may be used for suspension alone or for suspension and compression. When it is used for suspension alone, the patient rests in the sling and is suspended as in a hammock; when used for suspension and compression, the ends of the sling are drawn toward the midline over the patient, compressing the pelvis. The compression force is controlled by adjusting the distance between the ends of the sling on the spreader bar (Fig. 7-7). The physician determines the amount of compression. Suspension always remains the same, just barely touching the mattress.

Draw the ends of the sling toward the midline over the patient, compressing the pelvis. Control the compression force by adjusting the distance between the edges of the sling on

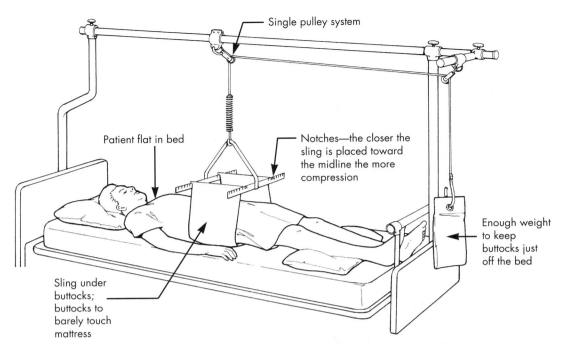

Single pulley system

Patient flat in bed

Notches—the closer the sling is placed toward the midline the more compression

Enough weight to keep buttocks just off the bed

Sling under buttocks; buttocks to barely touch mattress

Figure 7-7   The pelvic sling.

the spreader bar. The physician determines the amount of compression and suspension needed.

Mechanical Components

Angles. The patient lies flat in bed with a pillow under the head.

Weights. Enough weight is attached to allow the buttocks to barely touch the mattress.

Pulleys. The sling is suspended from a spreader bar, which is suspended from a single overhead pulley.

Countertraction. Countertraction is provided by the weight of the patient.

RELATED NURSING DIAGNOSES (PELVIC SLING AND PELVIC TRACTION)

Impaired Physical Mobility: Related to bedrest and traction application

Assessment	Rationale
Assess skin integrity on admission to hospital	May need to change treatment plan if open areas are present or if skin is otherwise compromised
Assess alignment of body	For traction to function properly, patient must lie straight in bed
Check for proper application of pelvic belt and straps and pelvic sling	Indicates that pull prescribed by physician is in place; also decreases risk of skin breakdown and pain
Assess for appropriate line of pull	Indicates that appropriate traction is being applied

Assessment	Rationale		Assessment	Rationale
Assess neurological status	Patients treated in this type of traction may have injuries or conditions that predispose to neurological deficits		Assess skin integrity on admission to hospital	May need to change treatment plan if open areas are present or skin is otherwise compromised
Assess ability to perform ADLs	If traction is intermittent, patient may be able to perform some ADLs independently		Assess patient's complaints of discomfort	May indicate area of concern not evident on examination (i.e., DVT)
			Assess lower extremity for swelling	May indicate complication (e.g., DVT)
			Assess nutritional status and hydration	Malnourished (depleted protein stores) or dehydrated patient is at increased risk of skin breakdown
			Assess mental status	Confused or agitated patient is prone to skin breakdown resulting from excessive movement, incontinence, and noncompliance
			Assess all skin that comes in contact with pelvic sling or pelvic straps at least every 2 to 3 hours	Decreases risk of skin breakdown
				Potential skin problems may be recognized and treated immediately
			Inspect used linens and change as needed	Changing soiled linen in timely manner decreases risk of breakdown

Interventions

1. Patients in pelvic traction may be turned and repositioned every 2 hours if allowed.

2. Teach the patient in pelvic tracdtion how to get out of bed without increasing discomfort or risking further injury.

   a. Remove the pelvic sling or belt.

   b. Instruct the patient to turn to either side.

   c. Tell the patient to use his hands to push the upper body up in one smooth straight motion while simultaneously swinging the legs over the side of the bed.

   d. Stand at the side of the bed toward which the patient will be getting up so you will be in front of the patient when he is sitting on the edge of the bed.

   e. When returning the patient to bed in the pelvic belt, make sure that the straps are in the configuration that the physician ordered.

3. Encourage the patient to do as much self-care as possible.

4. Encourage participation in an exercise program to maintain muscle tone, strength, and motion in the extremities.

NOTE: Patients treated with a pelvic sling are usually not allowed to turn or get out of bed.

Alteration in Skin Integrity: Related to traction application and immobility.

Interventions

1. Keep the skin clean and dry.

2. Inspect the skin for redness, cyanosis, blistering, increased temperature, and circulation at least every 2 to 3 hours.

3. Avoid pressure on bony prominences and other areas.

4. Turn and position the patient every 2 hours if tolerated.

5. Massage the coccyx and scapulae with a lubricant to keep the skin supple.

6. Massage the heels, elbows, and areas of the lower extremities.

7. Alleviate excessive pressure on the skin by using a special mattress or sheepskin, positioning the patient with pillows, applying special protectors (heel and elbow), or placing the patient on a therapeutic bed.

8. Avoid using a "donut" or rubber ring; these appliances restrict the circulation to the coccyx and increase the risk of skin breakdown.

9. Encourage the patient to follow a diet that provides adequate protein and calories.

10. Encourage adequate fluid intake to prevent dehydration. For a patient without medical restrictions, the suggested total intake is approximately 2600 ml per 24 hours.

11. Reinforce orientation as to time, place, and self if necessary.

12. Encourage family members to bring in familiar objects and pictures.

13. Keep a small night light on.

Pain: Related to fracture or injury and immobility

Assessment	Rationale
Assess for signs and symptoms of pain or discomfort in pelvis, back, or lower extremity	May indicate inappropriate treatment or improperly applied traction
	Indicates need to offer or administer analgesics
NOTE: Patients treated with pelvic sling may have more serious injury; it is therefore necessary to observe for injury to pelvic organs as well as for bladder injury and bleeding into pelvic area from injury to major vessels	May indicate complication (e.g., DVT)

Interventions

1. Administer analgesics as ordered.

2. Document the patient's response to the medication.

3. Teach the patient alternative methods of pain control to augment the use of analgesics, including guided imagery and relaxation techniques.

4. Encourage diversional activities.

5. Encourage visits by family and friends.

6. Turn and reposition the patient as needed.

Self-Care Deficits: Related to immobility and pain or position

Assessment	Rationale
Assess for ability to perform ADLs	Needed to determine level of activity; specifically, does patient require help with feeding, bathing, or toileting?

Interventions

1. Assist the patient with self-care activities as necessary.

2. Encourage the patient to do as much self-care as possible.

3. Position necessary equipment within reach.

High Risk for Peripheral Vascular Dysfunction: Related to injury and immobilization

Assessment	Rationale
Assess neurovascular status	Recognition of deficits allows early intervention

Interventions

To assess vascular status:

1. Check the presence and quality of pulses in the lower extremities.

2. Check capillary filling; use the blanching sign, which evaluates arterial return. Gently pinch the skin or nail bed of the lower extremity(ies). The nail bed or skin should "blanch" or turn white; then, as soon as the pressure of the pinch is eliminated, the area should return to its normal pink color. The rapidity with which this occurs demonstrates the presence or absence of capillary refill. If the skin does not return to its normal color within 2 to 4 seconds, suspect damage to the arterial circulation. Document and report these findings to the physician immediately.

3. Observe for swelling, warmth, and color of the legs. The extremities should be warm to the touch and the color about the same in both legs. If the leg(s) is cool to the touch and the nail beds have a whitish blue appearance, vascular integrity may be compromised.

To assess neurological status:

1. Ask the patient if he or she is experiencing any pain, numbness, tingling, or loss of sensation in the legs. Check for loss of sensation by touching the leg lightly with the hand or an open paper clip (being careful not to break the skin).

2. Check for continued motor function. Ask the patient to move both feet and legs.

3. Ask if the patient can feel gentle pressure exerted on a point distal to (below) the injury or traction application site.

4. Document your findings and notify the physician immediately of any abnormality or deficit in these areas.

▼

CARE GUIDE
CERVICAL HALTER TRACTION

The following information should be used in conjunction with the information found in the general traction management guide (Chapter 3).

MECHANICAL COMPONENTS

1. Weights . . . .
   a. Not more than 5 pounds for continuous traction
   b. Ten to 15 pounds for intermittent traction (10 to 15 minutes)

2. Pulleys . . . .
   a. Single-pulley system
   b. Pull is in straight line
   c. See general traction management guide (Chapter 3)

3. Ropes . . . .
   a. See general traction management guide (Chapter 3)

4. Countertraction . . . .
   a. Head of bed elevated 6 inches by shock blocks, reverse Tredelenburg, or adjustable pulley
   b. Make sure knot is not up against pulley

5. Angles . . . .
   a. Straight line

6. Bed . . . .
   a. See general traction management guide (Chapter 3)

7. Trapeze . . . .
   a. **Do not use**

8. Halter . . . .
   a. Evenly centered on chin
   b. Pull is on chin and occiput, not throat
   c. No pressure from ropes on face
   d. Ears are free
   e. Spreader bar attached appropriately

PATIENT ALIGNMENT	a. Straight in bed b. Small pillow or bath blanket under head for comfort c. Knees slightly flexed for comfort d. Log-roll side to side e. If allowed out of bed, use soft collar as ordered
MAINTENANCE OF SKIN INTEGRITY	a. See general traction management guide (Chapter 3)
NEUROVASCULAR IMPAIRMENT	a. See general traction management guide (Chapter 3)
ALTERATION IN GAS EXCHANGE	a. See cervical traction guide (next page)
ALTERATION IN NUTRITIONAL STATUS	a. See general traction management guide (Chapter 3)
ALTERATION IN ELIMINATION	a. See general traction management guide (Chapter 3)
INEFFECTIVE COPING	a. See general traction management guide (Chapter 3)

▼

CARE GUIDE
SKELETAL CERVICAL TRACTION

The following information should be used in conjunction with the information found in the general traction management guide (Chapter 3).

MECHANICAL COMPONENTS

1. Weights . . . .
   a. Prescribed by doctor
   b. Up to 35 pounds for reduction
   c. Secured
   d. Hanging freely
   e. See general traction management guide (Chapter 3)

2. Pulleys . . . .
   a. One-pulley system
   b. Pull is in straight line
   c. See general traction management guide (Chapter 3)

3. Ropes . . . .
   a. See general traction management guide (Chapter 3)

4. Countertraction . . . .
   a. Head of bed elevated 6 inches by shock blocks or reverse Trendelenburg
   b. Make sure knot is not up against pulley

5. Angles . . . .
   a. Straight line

6. Bed . . . .
   a. See general traction management guide (Chapter 3)

7. Trapeze . . . .
   a. **Do not use**

8. Cervical tongs . . . .
   a. Embedded in skull
   b. Check pin sites
   c. Tongs not pushing against pulley
   d. Tongs not pressing against scalp

9. Halo . . . .
     a. Pins embedded in skull
     b. Halo attached
     c. Rods in place
     d. Rods attached to jacket
     e. Check pin sites
     f. Pins not slipping
     g. Wrench for removal of vest readily available

PATIENT ALIGNMENT
     a. Straight in bed
     b. Small pillow or bath blanket under head for comfort
     c. Knees slightly flexed for comfort
     d. Log-roll patient side to side if ordered
     e. Support head and neck when turning

MAINTENANCE OF SKIN INTEGRITY
     a. See general traction management guide (Chapter 3)

NEUROVASCULAR IMPAIRMENT
     a. See general traction management guide

ALTERATION IN GAS EXCHANGE
     a. See general traction management guide
     b. Suction and oxygen readily available
     c. Tracheostomy set available

ALTERATION IN NUTRITIONAL STATUS
     a. See general traction management guide (Chapter 3)

ALTERATION IN ELIMINATION
     a. See general traction management guide (Chapter 3)

INEFFECTIVE COPING
     a. See general traction management guide (Chapter 3)

▼

CARE GUIDE
PELVIC TRACTION

The following information should be used in conjunction with the information found in the general traction management guide (Chapter 3).

MECHANICAL COMPONENTS

1. Weights . . . .   a. Should not exceed 8 to 10 pounds per strap

2. Pulleys . . . .   b. Two single-pulley systems, one to each strap

3. Ropes . . . .   c. See general traction management guide (Chapter 3)

4. Countertraction . . . .   d. Provided by weight of patient

5. Angles . . . .   e. Pull is in straight line
    (1) Along axis of femur
    (2) Patient remains in Williams position:
        (a) Hips and knees flexed 45 degrees
        (b) Lower legs parallel to floor
        (c) Head of bed elevated to 20 to 30 degrees

6. Bed . . . .   f. See general traction management guide (Chapter 3)

7. Pelvic belt . . . .   g. Placed just above and around iliac crests
    (1) Belt is correct size
    (2) Strap lengths are equal
    (3) Straps should clear bed

PATIENT ALIGNMENT

a. Williams position (see above)
b. In center of bed

NURSING CARE

a. See general traction management guide (Chapter 3)

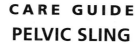

CARE GUIDE
PELVIC SLING

The following information should be used in conjunction with the information found in the general traction management guide (Chapter 3).

MECHANICAL COMPONENTS

1. Weights . . . . a. Prescribed by doctor
   (1) Enough to allow buttocks to barely touch mattress
   (2) See general traction management guide (Chapter 3)

2. Pulleys . . . . b. Single-pulley system on overhead frame

3. Ropes . . . . c. See general traction management guide (Chapter 3)

4. Countertraction . . . . d. Provided by weight of patient

5. Angles . . . . e. Patient lies flat with pillow under head

6. Bed . . . . f. See general traction management guide (Chapter 3)

7. Trapeze . . . . g. See general traction management guide (Chapter 3)

8. Sling . . . . h. Canvas sling placed under hips

9. Spreader bar . . . . i. Placed above sling, suspended by rope through pulley
   (1) Compression is accomplished by moving ends of sling toward midline of spreader bar
   (2) Doctor prescribes amount of compression

PATIENT ALIGNMENT
a. Flat in bed with pillow under head
b. Centered in bed

NURSING CARE
a. See general traction management guide (Chapter 3)

External Fixators

Another method of fracture management involves the use of an external fixator. This apparatus consists of pins placed at right or oblique angles into the bone and held by a frame using clamps and screws. Although it does not use the "traditional" traction components (ropes, pulleys, and weights), it does incorporate the principles of distraction, compression, reduction, and immobilization.

Fixators are usually applied by the physician in the operating room under sterile conditions. The area of pin insertion is prepared as for a surgical procedure. The physician may incise the skin for insertion of the pin or wire. A hand drill is then used to insert the pin or wire. Power drills are avoided because of the risk of bone injury. The high number of revolutions per minute produced by a power drill increases the risk of "burning" the bone and surrounding tissue, heightening the risk of infection.

There are three types of external fixation:

Type 1: Heavy pins drilled through the fractured bone and attached to the frame

Type 2: Small Kirschner wires drilled through the bone and attached to a circular metal ring

Type 3: Ilizarov fixation, employed primarily for leg-lengthening procedures

The external fixator can be used to treat fractures in the upper or lower extremity as well as fractures of the pelvis and mandible.

Some of its more common indications are as follows:

- Lower extremity
    Open fracture with soft tissue loss
    Segmental bone loss or comminution
    Nonunion
- Pelvis
    Open book fracture
    Lateral compression fracture
    Vertical shear fracture
- Upper extremity
    Unstable or open distal radius fracture
    Humerus fracture

Mechanical Components

Pins or wires: Two types of pins or wires are used for external fixation:

Transfixing pins, which are placed through the bone and may be smooth or threaded. These are avoided when the involved bone is surrounded by major blood vessels or nerves (Fig. 8-1).

Half pins, which do not transect the bone and can be entirely threaded or have an interrupted thread. These are used to avoid damaging surrounding tissue. (Usually more half pins than transfixing pins are needed to ensure rigid fixation or stabilization.) (Fig. 8-2).

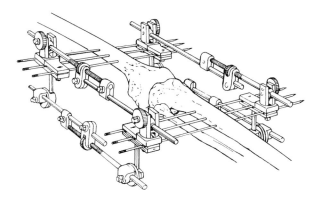

Figure 8-1   Transfixing pins used for external fixation.

Connecting rods: Solid connecting rods are included that are of appropriate length(s).

Clamps: Clamps are applied to the pins to accommodate the connecting rod(s).

The components used depend on the type and location of the fracture and the type of apparatus being employed. The various joints and bars of the frame allow adjustment of bone fragments during treatment, much as adjusting the weights, pulleys, and angles of a traction system allows for the manipulation of fracture fragments. This adjustability of pin angles accommodates alignment of the bone fragments and decreases the risk of malunion.

The ability to adjust the frame can facilitate

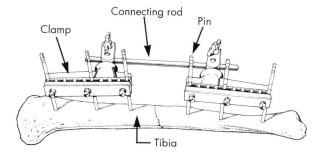

Figure 8-2   External fixation.

compression of a transverse fracture, maintenance of length in a comminuted fracture, or distraction of fragments in a simple fracture.

Advantages

- Allows the use of adjacent joints while maintaining fracture reduction, immobilization, and stability.
- Allows for early ambulation and therefore possibly earlier discharge.
- Allows for active treatment of soft tissue injuries, since wound is not enclosed in a cast.
- Can decrease the incidence of complications resulting from disuse or immobility.
- Can allow for separate and independent treatment of each site where fractures exist at more than one level.
- Decreases risk of sepsis by allowing free access for wound care and reducing need for internal fixation.
- May reduce blood loss by decreasing time in the operating room and limiting the size of the operative wound.

Disadvantages

- Not generally recommended for treatment of severely comminuted fractures when fragments lack good alignment. Exception: use of the Ilizarov external fixator, which allows for correction of three-dimensional deformities, including angulation, translation (lateral or sideways movement of the fracture surfaces in relation to each other), rotation, shortening, widening, lengthening, and soft tissue defects.
- Risk of pin site infection increased.
- May increase the risk of osteomyelitis.
- Possible pin loosening and movement with overuse or excessive movement.

- Once pins are removed, possible bone weakness, increasing the risk of refracture.
- Possible damage to nerves, blood vessels, or muscle (muscle impingement) during insertion of the pin(s).
- Risk of cellulitis present.

Nursing Care of the Patient with an External Fixator on the Lower Extremity

RELATED NURSING DIAGNOSES

Impaired Physical Mobility: Related to injury

Assessment	Rationale
Assess for swelling	Increased swelling may occur when patient is out of bed
Assess for ability to ambulate	Weight-bearing status must be ordered before ambulation begins
Assess for position of extremity	Avoid pressure on peroneal nerve
Assess patient's ability to care for pins and apparatus	May increase independence and self-esteem

Interventions

1. Keep the extremity on pillows or in balanced suspension (Thomas splint) to maintain elevation. Alternatively, attach a traction rope to four locations on the fixator frame, running the ropes through pulleys attached to the overhead frame. **Do not attach the ropes to the pins.** This can lead to pin bending, or the pin may cut through the skin.

2. Make sure that the foot remains in a neutral position until the patient can dorsiflex it.

3. To minimize the risk of peroneal nerve damage, avoid external rotation of the limb.

4. Encourage the patient to be up in a chair if allowed.

5. Encourage ambulation with assistance if ordered.

6. Monitor the patient while ambulating to assure proper gait, weight-bearing status, and use of assistive devices.

7. Instruct the patient to be aware of the pins so injury to the unaffected extremity will be avoided. To decrease this risk, use pin covers (e.g., corks, Vacutainer vial plugs, rubber Tubex needle covers, or commercial plastic covers).

Alteration in Skin Integrity: Related to immobility and pin insertion

Assessment	Rationale
Assess pin sites for redness, swelling, purulent drainage, tenting of skin, increased temperature or excessive crusting around pins	To decrease risk of pin site infection
Assess skin integrity on admission and every 4 to 8 hours as needed	May need to change treatment plan if open areas are present or skin integrity is compromised
Assess for neurovascular status	Immediate intervention is needed if neurovascular dysfunction is noted
Assess for swelling of extremity	May indicate development of compartment syndrome
Assess for nutritional status and hydration	Malnourished (depleted protein stores) or dehydrated patient is at increased risk of skin breakdown

Interventions

1. Provide pin site care according to hospital and physician protocol.

2. Encourage the patient to be up and about as soon as possible and to participate in range-of-motion (ROM) exercises.

3. Teach the patient to care for the pin sites as soon as possible.

4. To decrease the degree of swelling, keep the extremity elevated when the patient is sitting or lying in bed.

5. Make sure that the skin is kept dry and clean and that the sheets are unwrinkled.

6. Encourage the patient to eat a nutritionally balanced diet.

Pain: Related to injury and pin insertion

Assessment	Rationale
Assess for signs and symptoms of pain and discomfort	May indicate inappropriate treatment or improperly applied apparatus
	Indicates need to offer or administer analgesics
	May indicate complication (e.g., compartment syndrome)
Assess patient's ability to care for pins	Allows patient to be as independent as possible

Interventions

1. To facilitate activities of daily living (ADLs), encourage the patient to be out of bed as soon as possible.

2. Inform the patient that increased mobility increases the amount of swelling and drainage from the pin sites.

3. Teach the patient to get back in bed or to sit in a chair and elevate the extremity to decrease these occurrences..

4. Teach the patient pin site care .

5. Caution the patient about injury to the

unaffected extremity from the pins. Wearing long trousers on the unaffected leg may help to decrease the risk of injury, as will covering the pin ends with appropriate caps.

6. Teach the patient to use the trapeze to facilitate movement.

High Risk for Neurovascular Dysfunction: Related to pin placement

Assessment	Rationale
Assess for motion and sensation of peroneal and tibial nerves	If neurovascular impairment is recognized, appropriate interventions may decrease sequelae
Assess for color, temperature, pulses, and blanching	Needed to detect problems in vascular status

Interventions

1. Test for sensation and motion of the peroneal and tibial nerves:

- **Peroneal nerve**
  Sensation: Touch the web space between the patient's great toe and second toe; decreased sensation may indicate nerve pressure
  Motion: Have the patient dorsiflex the ankle and extend the toes (similar to stepping on a car's brake pedal); inability to perform this function may indicate nerve impairment
- **Tibial nerve**
  Sensation: Touch the sole of the patient's foot along the medial and lateral aspects; decreased sensation may indicate nerve impairment
  Motion: Have the patient plantarflex the ankle (point the toes downward); inability to do this may indicate nerve impairment

2. Perform neurovascular checks at least every hour immediately after surgery. Decrease

frequency to every 2 to 4 hours as the patient's condition stabilizes.

Care of the Patient with an External Fixator on the Pelvis

Fractures of the pelvis can be treated with an external fixator. Most often the pins are drilled into the iliac crests and the frame is attached anteriorly.

RELATED NURSING DIAGNOSES

Impaired Physical Mobility: Related to injury and pin insertion

Assessment	Rationale
Assess patient's ability to move in bed and get out of bed	May need extra help in performing these activities
Assess patient for appropriate method of ambulation and weight-bearing status	May need instruction in use of assistive devices
Assess for movement of pins	Movement of frame may cause movement of pins
Assess skin integrity	Movement of pins can cause pin site infection

Interventions

1. Provide pin site care according to hospital and physician protocol.
2. Avoid pulling on the frame when moving the patient.
3. Turn the patient if tolerated.
4. Position the patient on pillows for comfort.
5. Protect abdominal skin when turning, especially if the patient is obese.
6. Encourage the patient to sit in a chair as soon as tolerated.

7. Encourage ambulation using suitable assistive devices and appropriate gait pattern.
8. Be aware that increased movement caused by ambulation may increase the risk of pin loosening, pin site drainage or infection, and skin breakdown.
9. Document your findings and report any signs of the above immediately.

Pain: Related to injury and pin insertion

Assessment	Rationale
Assess for signs of DVT and thrombophlebitis	DVT is common complication after pelvic injury
Assess for signs and symptoms of pain	Indicate need to offer or administer analgesics; may also indicate need to change method of treatment

Interventions

1. Monitor the patient's vital signs and neurovascular status.
2. Be aware of the signs and symptoms of DVT.
3. Administer appropriate analgesics.
4. Encourage alternative methods of pain control (e.g., relaxation techniques and guided imagery).

High Risk for Neurovascular Dysfunction: Related to injury and pin insertion

Assessment	Rationale
Assess sciatic and lateral cutaneous nerves	These are most commonly injured with insertion of pelvic pins
Assess general vascular function	Appropriate interventions in a timely fashion decrease risk of sequelae

The sciatic nerve runs deep in the gluteus maximus before passing under the piriformis muscle and then travels down the posterior aspect of the thigh. Injury to it can manifest as decreased knee flexion and loss of sensation on the lateral side of the leg and foot. The leg and foot can become edematous secondary to severe injury, with discoloration and vasomotor changes.

The lateral cutaneous nerve enters the thigh between the two attachments of the inguinal ligament and divides into two branches just below it. The anterior branch supplies sensation to the lateral portion of the anterior thigh as far as the knee. The posterior branch supplies the upper two thirds of the lateral thigh and lateral aspect of the buttock. If this nerve is injured during pin placement, the patient may complain of pain, paresthesias, or numbness in the area of distribution (i.e., lateral thigh and buttock).

Interventions

1. Monitor the neurovascular status of the lower extremities.

2. Check for numbness and tingling over the lateral aspect of the thigh and lower leg.

3. Monitor the patient's motion, flexion and extension of the knees, and pedal and popliteal pulses. Also note any swelling.

- Monitor the color and temperature of both extremities.
- Document your findings and notify the physician immediately if any of the above occur.

Alteration in Gas Exchange: Related to injury

Assessment	Rationale
Assess for signs of pulmonary embolism (PE)	PE can be a complication of pelvic fractures

Assessment	Rationale
Assess respiratory status for decreased breath sounds, rales or rhonchi, and wheezing	May indicate respiratory compromise or pneumonia
Assess vital signs, including temperature, pulse, and respirations	Alterations may indicate respiratory compromise

Interventions

1. Monitor vital signs. Document your findings and report any changes.

2. Encourage the patient to be out of bed and to report any chest pain, coughing, epistaxis, or shortness of breath.

3. Be aware of subtle changes in mental status.

Ineffective Coping: Related to injury and pin placement

Assessment	Rationale
Assess ability to wear appropriate clothing	Placement of pins makes this difficult
Assess for problems associated with altered body image	Watch for signs of withdrawal and make appropriate referrals

Interventions

1. Allow the patient to talk freely about feelings regarding the pelvic frame.

2. Encourage the patient and family to participate in care of the frame and pin sites. This increases their self-esteem and decreases the patient's anxiety regarding the frame and pins.

3. Access the appropriate resources (social service, psychological service, pastoral service, etc.) as needed.

4. Encourage friends and family to visit, but allow time for the patient to be alone.

5. Encourage diversional activities.

Care of the Patient with an External Fixator on the Upper Extremity

RELATED NURSING DIAGNOSES

Impaired Physical Mobility: Related to injury

Assessment	Rationale
Assess ROM of adjacent joints	Prevents contractures and limitation of movement
Assess patient's ability to ambulate	Fixator may create sensation of imbalance

Interventions

1. Encourage the patient to be out of bed as much as possible.

2. To decrease swelling, support the arm in a sling when the patient is up and about.

3. Encourage the patient to move the adjacent joints as tolerated, putting the joints through a range of motion.

4. Encourage the patient to participate in a program of active exercise to provide finger extension and flexion and active movement of the elbow and shoulder.

Alteration in Skin Integrity: Related to injury and pin placement

See section on lower extremity (p. 104).

Pain: Related to injury

See section on lower extremity (p. 105).

Self-care Deficit: Related to injury and pin placement

Assessment	Rationale
Assess for ability to perform ADLs	If dominant extremity is affected, patient may require assistance
Assess for possible need for assistive devices	If patient's balance is impaired, such device (e.g., cane) may be required

Interventions

1. Monitor the patient's ability to provide self-care and assist as necessary.

2. Encourage the patient to be out of bed as much as possible. Provide support for the affected extremity.

3. Monitor the patient's ability to ambulate safely.

4. Provide assistive devices as needed.

5. Teach the patient or significant other to provide pin site care.

6. Access appropriate resources for home care.

Alteration in Neurovascular Status: Related to pin placement

Assessment	Rationale
Assess for motion and sensation of radial, ulnar, and median nerves	May be injured during pin placement

Interventions

1. Monitor the motion and sensation of the following nerves:

- Radial nerve
  Sensation: Touch the space between the thumb and index finger. If decreased sensation is demonstrated, the radial nerve may be impaired.
  Motion: Have the patient extend the thumb, wrist, and fingers from the metacarpophalangeal joints (knuckles) as far as possible. If unable to extend the thumb, wrist, and fingers, the radial nerve may be impaired.
- Ulnar nerve
  Sensation: Touch the distal fat pad of the little finger. If the patient is unable to feel this, ulnar nerve impairment may be suspected.
  Motion: Have the patient spread the fingers apart. If he is unable to do so, ulnar nerve entrapment may be suspected.

- Median nerve
  Sensation: Touch the distal surface of the index finger. If the patient is unable to feel this, it may indicate median nerve impairment.
  Motion: Have the patient put the thumb and little finger together and flex the wrist. If he is unable to perform either of these acts, median nerve impairment may be present.

2. Monitor and document the neurovascular status of the extremity at least every 2 hours until the patient's condition is stable.

3. Notify the physician immediately if there is any deficit or the patient complains of extreme pain or pain on motion, especially passive motion.

4. Notify the physician immediately if increased swelling is detected, the extremity is pale or bluish, or you find decreased pulses.

5. Keep the extremity elevated.

6. Encourage movement (ROM of the fingers).

Alteration in Gas Exchange

Ineffective Coping

For discussion of these topics, see sections on the lower extremity and pelvis (p. 107).

The Ilizarov External Fixator

The Ilizarov external fixator is gaining popularity in the United States. Devised in Russia, it is used to lengthen or widen bones and to correct angular or rotational defects of fractures and immobilization.

The Ilizarov fixator is similar to the conventional external fixators in that it consists of several Kirschner wires embedded in the bone and attached to a series of half or full rings around the affected extremity. The rings are then connected to each other using threaded or telescoping rods.

The Ilizarov fixator is used mainly for limb-lengthening procedures. The long bones (tibia, femur, humerus) grow only at the **growth plates**. Therefore lengthening the bone in an extremity that has stopped growing requires creation of a temporary or "false" growth plate. A corticotomy (an osteotomy through the cortex of the affected bone) is performed in the operating room when the pins for the fixator are inserted.

To lengthen the limb, the bone is distracted (pulled apart) in a controlled and consistent manner so the new bone forms without risking local ischemia, which slows bone formation. The usual distraction rate is 0.25 mm four times per day. Distraction is begun between the second and tenth days post surgery (depending on the patient's status, the condition of the limb, and the physician's preference). It is accomplished by turning the nuts that affix the frame to the rods. As the nuts turn, the rods lengthen and the bone ends are pulled apart.

When the desired length has been achieved, the distraction is discontinued. However, the apparatus is left in place until complete healing is documented on x-ray.

It may take several months to achieve the desired limb length. The patient and family must be aware of the time and commitment needed for a successful outcome.

RELATED NURSING DIAGNOSES

Pain: Related to pin insertion and operative procedure

Assessment	Rationale
Assess for signs and symptoms of pain	Indicates need to offer or administer analgesics

Assessment	Rationale
Assess for signs and symptoms of pain	May indicate complications (e.g., ischemia, thrombophlebitis, or compartment syndrome) May indicate increased anxiety

Interventions

1. Offer analgesics as ordered.

2. Monitor for signs and symptoms of thrombophlebitis or compartment syndrome.

3. Encourage the patient to verbalize feelings.

4. Offer reassurance.

5. Encourage the patient to participate in the distraction process.

Alteration in Mobility: Related to the fixator

Assessment	Rationale
Assess for ability to ambulate	Need to determine how much assistance the patient will require
Assess for ability to perform ADLs	Need to determine how much assistance the patient will require

Interventions

1. Provide appropriate assistive devices. The patient may be partially weight bearing initially and, once healing has occurred, may be allowed to bear full weight even while still in the apparatus. Encourage this progression.

2. Assist the patient with activities of daily living (ADLs) as needed.

3. Encourage the patient to perform as many activities as possible.

Ineffective Coping: Related to presence of the fixator

Assessment	Rational
Assess for signs of withdrawal or decreased interest in self-care	May indicate that patient is becoming depressed May indicate need to access supportive resources
Assess patient's support group	Visits by family and friends can help patient get well and maintain motivation

Interventions

1. Allow the patient to ventilate feelings.

2. Encourage the patient to be out of bed as much as tolerated.

3. Encourage family and friends to visit.

4. Encourage self-care as much as possible.

5. Encourage the patient and family to take an active role in caring for the pins, the apparatus, and the distraction process.

CARE GUIDE
EXTERNAL FIXATORS

The following information should be used in conjunction with the information found in the general traction management guide (Chapter 3).

MECHANICAL COMPONENTS

1. Pins and wires . . . .
   a. Transfixing pins (placed through bone)
   b. Half pins (one on each side)
   c. Should be straight, not pressing on skin or bowed

2. Connecting rods . . . .
   a. Solid rods of appropriate lengths, straight

3. Clamps . . . .
   a. Appropriately placed on pins and attached to connecting rods

4. Bed . . . .
   a. Firm mattress
   b. Siderails
   c. Trapeze
   d. See general traction management guide (Chapter 3)

PATIENT ALIGNMENT

1. If suspension is used . . . .
   a. Suspension apparatus is freely movable so it moves with patient
   b. All necessary items are within reach of patient
   c. Ropes are attached to fixator frame, **not** to pins
   d. Ropes ride freely over pulley(s)
   e. Knots tied to prevent slipping

2. Position of extremity . . . .
   a. Foot kept in neutral position
   b. Avoid external rotation

MAINTENANCE OF SKIN INTEGRITY

1. Check pressure points . . . .   a. Assess bony prominences

2. Adjunct equipment . . . .   a. Special mattress (avoid water mattresses)

3. Potential for injury from exposed pins . . . . .   a. Pin covers in place

EVALUATION OF AFFECTED EXTREMITY

1. Alteration in tissue perfusion . . . .   a. Check pulses distal to injury
                                                                b. Check capillary filling
     c. Observe for warmth, color, and swelling

2. Alteration in neurological status . . . .   a. Assess for motion and sensation
         (1) Lower extremity
                (a) Peroneal nerve
                (b) Tibial nerve
         (2) Upper extremity
                (a) Radial nerve
                (b) Median nerve
                (c) Ulnar nerve
         (3) Pelvis
                (a) Sciatic nerve
                (b) Lateral cutaneous nerve

3. Potential for pin site infection . . . .   a. Observe pin sites for redness, increased warmth, edema, pain, prolonged drainage, purulent drainage
     b. Observe for tenting of skin and/or excessive crusting around pin sites
     c. Observe for loosening of pins
     d. Make sure patient is receiving prescribed pin site care

ALTERATION IN SELF-CARE

a. Assess patient's ability to participate in self-care and encourage self-care within limits of ability

b. Instruct patient and significant other in pin site care

c. Patient and significant other should give satisfactory return demonstration of pin site care

d. Make sure that patient understands signs and symptoms of pin site infection

e. Have patient verbalize understanding of care and management of external fixator

f. Advise patient on how to make adaptation to clothing if necessary

ALTERATION IN GAS EXCHANGE

a. Monitor vital signs and respirations q2h immediately postoperatively

b. Encourage patient to be out of bed

c. Have patient cough and deep breathe

ALTERATION IN ELIMINATION

a. Monitor urinary output

b. Monitor bowel function

c. Assess for any evidence of bleeding

ALTERATION IN COMFORT

a. Keep extremity elevated

b. Medicate as necessary

c. Monitor for complications (e.g., compartment syndrome)

INEFFECTIVE COPING

a. Allow patient to verbalize

b. Encourage involvement of family

c. Investigate home and family situation to assess need for intervention (discharge planning)

d. Make referrals to appropriate services as needed

9

Major Complications: Prevention, Recognition, and Nursing Care

Complications may occur in any patient being treated in traction. Most of these complications are not directly associated with the traction apparatus but may be attributed to the prolonged bedrest imposed on the patient or to the extent of the injury being treated. The complications that will be addressed in this chapter are

1. Deep vein thrombosis (DVT)
2. Pulmonary embolism (PE)
3. Fat embolism syndrome (FES)
4. Compartment syndrome
5. Peroneal nerve palsy and footdrop
6. Pin site infection

Deep Vein Thrombosis (DVT)

One of the most common complications associated with immobility is DVT. There are three terms with which the nurse must be familiar when discussing DVT: "thrombus," "phlebitis," and "thrombophlebitis." In some instances these terms are erroneously used interchangeably; however, each has a distinct definition. A thrombus is a blood clot within a blood vessel. Phlebitis is the inflammation of the vein that may occur as a result of the clot formation.

Thrombophlebitis is the overall condition in which there is a clot with inflammation of the vein.

A clot can occur following a fracture as a result of damage to the vein wall secondary to the trauma. In addition, the immobility associated with traction increases the risk of venous stasis, which can result in clot formation. DVTs usually occur in the lower extremity.

The process of clot formation starts when the platelets come in contact with a damaged vein wall or the blood is allowed to pool in the vein secondary to lack of motion. As the platelets collect, they stick to the wall and a clot forms. The platelets become more permeable and finally rupture, releasing the clotting factors for fibrin formation. These fibrin strands then act to collect more blood cells and platelets, causing the formation of a larger clot and reducing the flow of blood out of the affected area.

The incidence of DVT has been reported to be as high as 45% to 70% in the orthopaedic population (patients with total joint replacements, hip fractures, or major knee reconstructions). This is greater than in the general surgical population.

The primary risk factors associated with the development of DVT are obesity, immobility, the presence of fractures, a prior history of DVT, age, a history of trauma, use of oral contraceptives, a history of heart disease, and a history of cigarette smoking.

Assessment	Rationale
Assess for risk factors	If above factors are present, prophylaxis may be started
Assess for presence and sites of fractures	Risk is increased in patient with lower extremity fracture or multiple injuries
Assess for signs and symptoms	Signs and symptoms include pain and tenderness along vein with swelling, redness, and increased skin temperature of extremity
Assess for Homan's sign	Positive Homan's sign may indicate thrombophlebitis

Assessing for Homan's sign. Although the diagnosis of DVT should not be based solely on this test, the results of the test must be considered. This test is controversial, and the nurse should use discretion when relying on it to verify the presence of DVT.

To assess for Homan's sign, instruct the patient to move his or her toes upward toward the head (dorsiflexion of the foot). This stretches the muscles, nerves, and vessels in the calf. If the patient complains of pain in the calf while performing this function, it is said that a positive Homan's sign has been elicited, which may indicate the presence of thrombophlebitis.

Interventions for Prevention

1. Encourage ambulation as soon as the patient is able to get out of bed.

2. Start a program of active and passive ROM exercises for the unaffected extremity when the patient must remain immobilized.

3. Make sure that the circulation in the affected extremity is not compromised by an ill-fitting or improperly applied traction apparatus.

4. Change the patient's position frequently. Turn the patient if possible, or have him or her lift for skin care. The patient may also be lifted for position changes. Skin assessment and exercise can be done at the same time.

5. Avoid use of the knee gatch, which allows blood to pool in the lower extremities.

6. Consider using elastic stockings or sequential compression boots on the unaffected leg to enhance peripheral circulation. Sequential compression boots should not be used on patients with severe peripheral vascular disease or those who have a history of compartment syndrome, because the boots may exacerbate these problems.

Prophylactic anticoagulation. If the patient is at high risk of developing thrombophlebitis, the physician may elect to administer an anticoagulant for prophylaxis. The most commonly used drugs are aspirin, heparin, and warfarin (Coumadin). The choice of drug is according to physician preference and depends on the rate of anticoagulation desired and the patient's condition.

Heparin is used for rapid anticoagulation and can be administered subcutaneously or intravenously. It prevents the conversion of prothrombin to thrombin, reaching a peak acting time in 2 to 4 hours. The dose ranges from 5000 to 10,000 units initially, followed by 5000 to 20,000 units IV every 4 to 12 hours. It can also be given by continuous intravenous infusion. Blood levels should indicate an activated partial thromboplastin time (PTT) of 1.5 to 2 times the normal level for adequate maintenance antico-agulation. The parameters set at each hospital differ, so you must check with the laboratory to ascertain the appropriate PTT levels.

Coumadin (warfarin) is an oral medication used for maintenance and long-term anticoag-ulation. It acts by interfering with the synthesis of vitamin K. Its peak level of action occurs 1 to 9 hours after administration, but the anticoag-ulation effect is not evident until 36 to 72 hours after the initial dose (which is usually 10 mg). Subsequent doses depend on the pro-thrombin time (PT) levels. The goal is to main-tain the PT at 1.5 to 2 times the control value. Again, each hospital is unique and these levels should be confirmed with the laboratory.

NOTE: Neither heparin nor warfarin (Coumadin) will dissolve an existing clot.

If the patient is undergoing anticoagulation therapy, be cognizant of the possibility of de-layed clotting. Observe for excessive bruising, bleeding from the gums, and blood in the urine or stool. If any of these signs or symp-toms are observed, notify the physician imme-diately. Common antidotes include protamine sulfate (1%) for heparin overdose and vitamin K for Coumadin.

High Risk for Alteration in Circulation: Related to the development of DVT

Assessment	Rationale
Assess for swelling, redness, increased pain in calf of affected extremity, and positive Homan's sign	All may indicate DVT or thrombophlebitis

Interventions

1. Encourage early ambulation.
2. Initiate active and passive ROM exercises as soon as possible.
3. Change the patient's position frequently,

encouraging him (or her) to assist as much as possible.

4. Avoid using the knee gatch.
5. Apply elastic stockings or use sequential compression boots if there is no history of se-vere peripheral vascular disease or compart-ment syndrome.
6. Administer anticoagulation medication as ordered.

Pulmonary Embolism (PE)

A pulmonary embolism (PE) is a clot that has traveled from the systemic circulation (possibly a lower extremity DVT) into the pulmonary cir-culation, where it obstructs one or both branches of the pulmonary artery (Fig. 9-1). When a clot forms in the peripheral circula-tion, it may become dislodged and migrate through the venous system until it reaches the right side of the heart, where it may enter the lung via the pulmonary artery and cause an ob-struction. The obstruction can lead to pul-monary infarction, right-side heart failure, and death.

The incidence of clinically significant PEs may be as high as 20% in patients undergoing hip surgery, 1% to 3% of which are fatal. The risk factors associated with PE are similar to those for DVT. A pulmonary embolism usually occurs within 48 to 72 hours of injury or surgery.

Signs and symptoms of PE vary with the size and number of clots present. They may be vague or sudden, leading to immediate death.

Assessment	Rationale
Assess for signs of PE: Unexplained fever Worsening of pre-existing cardiac or cardiopulmonary condition	If subtle signs are recognized, prophy-laxis can be initiated

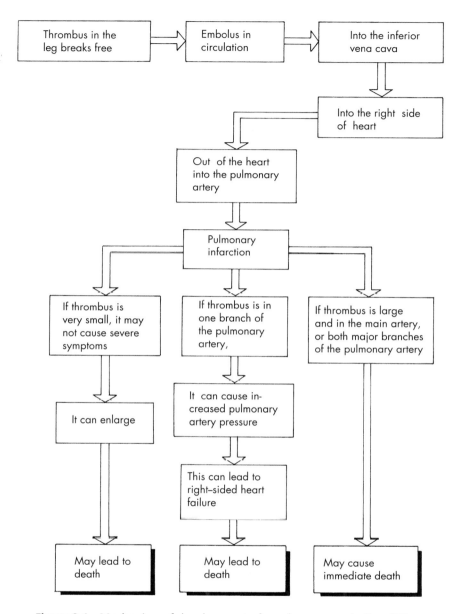

Figure 9-1   Mechanism of development of a pulmonary embolism (PE).

Assessment	Rationale
Assess for other signs and symptoms: Pleuritic chest pain Friction rub Hemoptysis Fever Dyspnea, cyanosis Tachypnea, tachycardia Restlessness, apprehension, confusion, decreased level of consciousness (LOC) shock Vital signs	Diagnostic tests can be ordered to document presence, number, and location of PEs and interventions initiated

Interventions

1. In addition to oxygen and fluid replacement, anticoagulation medication such as heparin and Coumadin will be ordered. (See section on DVT, above.)

2. Thrombolytic therapy (i.e., administration of urokinase or streptokinase) may be initiated. However, this is generally avoided in patients who have recently suffered major traumatic injuries or have undergone major surgery, because the risk of hemorrhage is increased.

3. Surgical treatments, including the insertion of various filters and the actual removal of the embolus (i.e., a pulmonary embolectomy), may be employed.

RELATED NURSING DIAGNOSES (PE)

Pain: Related to swelling, inflammation, pleuritic chest pain.

Assessment	Rationale
Assess for behavioral changes: Moaning Crying	May indicate presence of a DVT or PE

Assessment	Rationale
Restlessness Withdrawal Guarding Grimacing	
Assess for alteration in muscle tone: Spasm Listlessness Rigid fixation of extremity	Will help to reach diagnosis (i.e., patient who is not willing or able to move extremity may have thrombophlebitis)
Assess for autonomic and systemic responses: Diaphoresis Change in blood pressure Change in respiration Pupillary dilation Chest pain Hemoptysis	Changes indicate possibility of PE

Interventions

1. Administer analgesics as ordered. If the physician has prescribed heparin or warfarin (Coumadin), the use of aspirin, aspirin products, and other nonsteroidal antiinflammatory medications (ibuprofen, naproxen) is contraindicated because of the increased risk of bleeding.

2. Monitor and document the effects of the medication.

3. Provide other modalities to augment pain relief (e.g., relaxation techniques, guided imagery, or diversional activities).

4. If a thrombophlebitis is suspected, apply warm moist compresses to the affected extremity.

5. Elevate the extremity on a pillow, if allowed, to enhance circulation. When moving the extremity, support the leg at the joints (knee and ankle), avoiding the muscle belly of the calf because pressure on this area increases pain.

Anxiety: Related to the threat of death, threat of altered self-concept, threat of altered role functioning, and situational crisis.

Assessment	Rationale
Assess for increased apprehension and stated fears of consequences	Patients experiencing PE may appear anxious and frightened before any physical changes
Assess for changes in blood pressure, pulse, respirations, pupillary dilation, restlessness, facial tension, voice quivering, focus on self, diaphoresis, and trembling	May be signs of PE

Interventions

1. Offer appropriate explanations in terms that the patient and significant other can understand.

2. Assist with relaxation techniques.

3. Administer medications as ordered.

4. Instruct the patients in anticoagulation therapy, risk factors, and exercise programs.

High Risk for Impaired Gas Exchange: Related to pulmonary embolism

Assessment	Rationale
Assess for confusion, somnolence, restlessness, irritability, inability to move secretions, hypercapnea, or hypoxemia	All are signs or symptoms of PE
Monitor any change in blood pressure, pulse, respirations, temperature; observe for cyanosis, apprehension, hemoptysis, and diaphoresis	May indicate PE

Interventions

1. Administer oxygen as ordered.

2. Assess the need for more appropriate forms of ventilation.

3. Elevate the head of the bed to 30 to 40 degrees if allowed.

4. Monitor arterial blood gases.

5. Offer adequate explanations to the patient and family or significant other.

6. Provide appropriate fluid replacement as ordered.

7. Provide appropriate analgesia as ordered.

Fat Embolism Syndrome

Fat emboli are globules of fat deposited in the bloodstream that migrate into the pulmonary circulation or to the brain. Fat embolism syndrome (FES) is the pulmonary insufficiency commonly associated with them.

Fat emboli are usually associated with multiple fractures and crush injuries. Although their exact pathophysiology is unknown, several theories exist. One is that the globules are released into the circulation from the bone marrow of a fractured bone. Another is that free fatty acids and neutral fats are released after trauma and these lead to platelet aggregation and fat globule formation. What is known for certain is that fat is deposited in the capillaries of the lungs and causes a pulmonary disorder similar to acute respiratory distress syndrome (ARDS).

Most fat emboli occur within 24 to 48 hours of an injury or manipulation of the fracture. The patient is usually a young male (20 to 40 years) because of the high incidence of trauma among this age group. However, fat emboli can occur at any age and in either sex.

Treatment modalities for FES include mechanical ventilation to combat hypoxemia and maintain adequate ventilation, IV fluid replacement to maintain adequate volume, and administration of steroids to help reduce the inflammatory process that accompanies FES.

Assessment	Rationale
Assess for changes in neurological status	Will help to make diagnosis (i.e., restlessness, confusion, and agitation)
Assess respiratory status	Will help to make diagnosis (i.e., dyspnea, tachypnea, rales, and wheezing)
Assess for changes in skin	Will help to make diagnosis (i.e., petechiae on chest, axillae, clavicular fossae, soft palate, conjunctivae, flanks, and abdomen)
Assess for changes on chest roentgenogram	Classical sign is "snow storm" effect because of fat globules in lungs

Interventions

1. Maintain fracture alignment and immobilization. Avoid moving the fractured extremity. If movement is absolutely necessary, be sure to maintain adequate support of the fracture site by splinting the extremity.
2. Monitor vital signs.
3. Administer medications and intravenous fluids as ordered.
4. Monitor respiratory status and maintain adequate ventilation.
5. Provide emotional support to the patient and family, especially if mechanical ventilation is needed.

RELATED NURSING DIAGNOSES (FES)

Impaired Gas Exchange: Related to fat globules in the pulmonary circulation

Assessment	Rationale
Assess for apprehension	Will help to identify classic signs (dyspnea, tachypnea, rales, wheezing, air hunger, cyanosis, and petechiae)

Interventions

1. Administer oxygen as ordered.
2. Provide adequate explanation to the patient and family or significant other, especially regarding the possibility of mechanical ventilation. Offer reassurance and support.
3. Monitor behavioral changes and level of consciousness.
4. Monitor arterial blood gases.

Anxiety: Related to fear of the unknown, fear of death, fear of the possibility of mechanical ventilation, and fear of the inability to communicate needs

Assessment	Rationale
Assess for apprehension, alterations in vital signs, restlessness, irritability, or confusion	May indicate FES

Interventions

1. Provide adequate explanations to the patient and family or significant other.
2. Provide support and stay with the patient and family or significant other if possible.
3. Develop a method of communication to be used during mechanical ventilation.

Alteration in Comfort: Related to chest pain

Assessment	Rationale
Assess for signs and symptoms of pain: Irritability Apprehension	May indicate FES

Assessment	Rationale
Guarding	May indicate FES
Moaning	
Diaphoresis	
Assess for alteration in vital signs	Changes may indicate FES

Interventions

1. Provide adequate analgesics as ordered.
2. Provide support and stay with the patient.

Compartment Syndrome

Compartment syndrome is a condition in which increased pressure within a limited space (e.g., a muscle compartment) compromises the circulation and function of the tissues within that space. Acute compartment syndrome often results from trauma and can be caused by external forces (constrictive dressings, casts, or traction) or by internal forces (bleeding into the compartment, effusion, crush injuries, or fractures).

The pathophysiology of compartment syndrome begins with an injury to a muscle compartment that is covered by an unyielding fibrous membrane called the fascia. Because the fascia supports and contains the muscles, swelling of the injured tissue results in tissue ischemia. The vessels dilate, causing the capillary pressure to increase and allowing more fluid to leave the capillary than enter. The ischemic muscles release histamine, which increases the permeability of the capillary wall and allows plasma protein to be released into the interstitial fluid. Because this creates an imbalance between the intravascular and interstitial pressures, the fluid cannot be resorbed by the capillary. This leads to an accumulation of fluid in the tissues, and increased intramuscular pressure, which causes compression of the small veins and arteries. Blood flow decreases,

leading to more ischemia and perpetuating the cycle. If the events are allowed to continue for more than 6 hours, irreversible neuromuscular damage can occur. If they are allowed to continue for 24 to 48 hours, the extremity may become paralyzed and useless. Compartment syndrome can develop immediately or up to 6 days after an injury (Fig. 9-2).

Compartment syndrome can occur at any age and usually affects the lower extremity. Many complications occur as a result—including hypoesthesia, motor weakness, infection, contracture of the affected extremity, renal failure, and death.

Signs and symptoms include pain that is progressive and out of proportion to what is anticipated. Pain will also occur on passive stretching of the affected muscle compartment. Paresthesias occur, and the extremity appears pale. There may be swelling, and the skin will appear taut and shiny. Pulses may or may not be present.

Therapeutic modalities include decreasing the pressure by removal of constricting bandages, casts, or traction. In some instances a fasciotomy may be indicated to release compartment pressure. Fasciotomy is the surgical incision and division of the fascia that covers, supports, and separates the muscles. If it is done, the surgical wound is often left open and unsutured until the tissue swelling subsides. During this period, assessment for and prevention of infection are extremely important. After tissue swelling has subsided, the surgeon returns the patient to the operating room to suture the fasciotomy. However, compartment syndrome can redevelop after suturing.

Assessment	Rationale
Assess for pain on passive motion	Classical sign of compartment syndrome

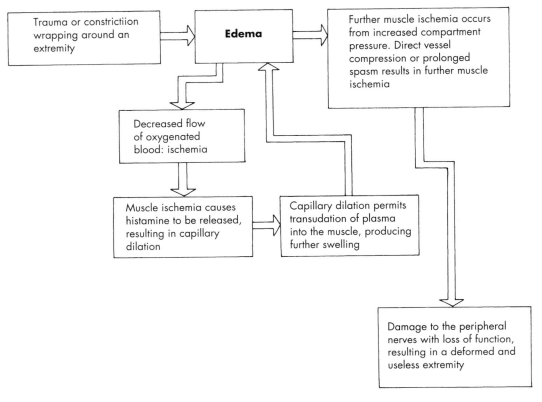

Figure 9-2 Compartment syndrome.

Assessment	Rationale
Assess for pallor, pulse-lessness, hypoesthesia, decreased muscle strength, tightness of compartment area, or tightness of bandage or cast	Any of these signs or symptoms indicate need to remove constrictive bandage or cast and report possibility of compartment syndrome to physician

RELATED NURSING DIAGNOSES (COMPARTMENT SYNDROME)

Potential for Renal Failure: Related to myoglobinuria

Myoglobinuria most commonly occurs if compression of the compartment is prolonged. The damaged muscle releases myoglobin into the circulation, which is then filtered into the kidneys. Renal failure may be secondary to the toxic effect of the myoglobin itself, renal vasoconstriction, or the presence of myoglobin within the renal tubules.

Assessment	Rationale
Assess for decreased urinary output	May indicate acute renal failure
Assess for alteration in vital signs	

Interventions

1. Increase fluid intake to maintain urinary output and dilute the effects of myoglobin on the kidneys.

2. Monitor IV intake.

3. Keep the urine alkaline by administration of either lactate or bicarbonate as ordered to minimize myoglobin precipitation.

Potential for Infection: Related to fasciotomy

Assessment	Rationale
Assess for signs and symptoms of infection: Increased temperature Purulent drainage Tissue necrosis	Indicate need to institute therapeutic measures

Interventions

1. Maintain sterility of all open wounds.

2. Administer antibiotics as ordered.

3. Monitor vital signs.

4. Monitor wounds for the presence of purulent drainage and necrotic tissue.

5. Monitor wound cultures and other laboratory values (e.g., WBC, erythrocyte sedimentation rate [ESR]).

6. Maintain appropriate limb splinting.

Alteration in Comfort: Related to pain and anxiety

Assessment	Rationale
Assess for signs and symptoms of pain and anxiety	May indicate need to medicate patient

Interventions

1. Do not elevate the extremity higher than the heart.

2. Administer analgesics as ordered.

3. Provide alternative methods of pain relief (e.g., guided imagery, diversional activity, or relaxation techniques).

4. Allow the patient to verbalize and vent feelings.

5. Provide emotional support to the patient and family.

6. Provide adequate and appropriate explanations to patient and family.

Alteration in Body Image: Related to fasciotomy scar

Assessment	Rationale
Assess for inability to view body part	Indicates need to provide access to appropriate resources (e.g., psychological services)
Assess for inability to care for body part when appropriate Assess for feelings of hopelessness or powerlessness	

Interventions

1. Reinforce reasons for the fasciotomy.

2. Explain all procedures.

3. Assist the patient in learning to care for the affected extremity.

4. Access appropriate resources (social service, psychological or psychiatric counseling) to help the patient cope with the situation.

Peroneal Nerve Palsy and Footdrop

The superficial peroneal nerve lies close to the proximal end of the fibula just below the knee on the lateral aspect. Wrapping this area tightly or allowing the patient's lower extremity to remain externally rotated places pressure on the area and possibly on the peroneal nerve. A patient who is experiencing pressure on the peroneal nerve will complain of pain, numbness, and tingling on the anterior surface of the leg and dorsum of the foot. He or she may also be unable to extend the toes or dorsiflex the foot.

Peroneal nerve palsy can result from compartment syndrome, excessive traction on the sciatic or peroneal nerve, or trauma that interferes with nerve function (i.e., improper placement of a tibial pin for balanced-suspension traction), or from the actual surgical procedure. The presence of peroneal nerve palsy or footdrop can significantly affect the patient's ability to ambulate and may require bracing the extremity. Bracing may be needed only temporarily or may be permanent depending on the degree of nerve damage.

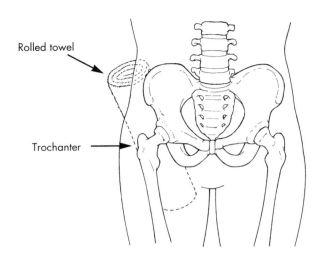

Figure 9-3   Proper position for trochanter roll.

Assessment	Rationale
Assess for proper position of extremity	If extremity is allowed to remain in external rotation, risk of pressure on or damage to peroneal nerve increases
Assess neurovascular status	Numbness, tingling, and inability to dorsiflex foot may indicate peroneal nerve involvement

Interventions

1. Maintain proper alignment of the affected extremity.

2. Avoid excessive pressure on the peroneal nerve by maintaining the lower extremity in neutral position. A trochanter roll can be used. This is made by rolling soft material, such as a bath blanket or towel, into a cylindrical shape 2 to 3 inches thick and 10 to 12 inches long. It is then placed under the greater trochanter on the affected side and rotates the trochanter

(and therefore the entire lower extremity) into neutral position. Proper placement is important. A patient with a fractured hip may not tolerate the positioning of a trochanter roll. In this instance, maintain the leg in neutral position by using pillows or folded bath blankets along the length of the leg. These must be removed periodically to check for pressure. Sandbags are not recommended because they can be an added source of pressure (Fig. 9-3).

Pin Site Infection

Pin site infection occurs at the points of entry and exit of a pin or wire used in skeletal traction or an external fixator. It can also occur at the site of insertion of tongs into the skull. Factors contributing to the incidence of pin site infection include movement of the pin (secondary to movement of the patient or to pin slippage), inadequate drainage of serous material following insertion of the pin or wire, improper insertion technique, and lack of sterility during insertion. An infection at the pin site can lead to the more serious condition of osteomyelitis (infection within the bone), because the pin or wire acts as a direct link to the bone.

Signs and symptoms of pin site infection include swelling, pain, redness, increased skin temperature, and purulent drainage.

Pin site infection is discussed in detail in Chapter 6.

10 Special Considerations

Patients admitted with multiple injuries may require treatment by various types of traction simultaneously. The person caring for these patients must possess appropriate nursing skills, a working knowledge of basic traction principles, creativity, and a good measure of common sense. The care involved in one type of traction may be contraindicated in another. For example, the patient in balanced-suspension traction for a fractured femur should be lifted for skin care. If he or she has also sustained a cervical fracture and is in cervical tong traction, then turning must be by log-rolling not lifting.

This predicament is often encountered in the intensive care setting, where you must consider many life support machines. Although life-threatening situations will take precedence over the treatment of fractures, orthopaedic management must not be compromised, because acute fracture management directly impacts on long-term outcome. Many innovations have been developed to maintain traction and immobilization while enabling the nurse to turn the patient and provide for basic needs.

Special beds have been available for years. The Stryker frame, a narrow, flat, wedge turning device, is used for patients who have sustained cervical vertebral injury. For turning,

the patient is sandwiched between the frames, which are secured by large steel pins at the head and foot and strapped together. The patient can be turned from the supine to the prone position, allowed to remain in the prone position for a set time, and then returned to the supine position. When in the desired position, the top frame may be removed. If done correctly, the spinal alignment remains undisturbed.

In caring for the patient in a Stryker frame, you must realize that turning may be a frightening experience for the patient. Explain the process and make sure the two frames are securely strapped together. In addition, before beginning the turn and before removing the top pins on either end of the frame after the turn, make sure the lower pins are securely in place. The turning must not disturb the traction or its line of pull.

The Stryker frame has been associated with numerous complications, especially when used with cervical traction. These include loss of reduction in the prone position from inadequate support of the chin, resulting in extension of the neck; loss of pulmonary vital capacity; and skin breakdown over the occiput. Because of these complications, because turning a patient on a Stryker frame produces pain at the fracture site, and because the frame cannot accommodate other types of traction, this method of treatment is rarely used today.

The Circ-O-Lectric bed also facilitates turning of the patient. It consists of a wide posterior frame and a narrow anterior frame, both of which are stabilized between two circular stands. It is used most often with patients who have sustained a stable cervical injury. As with the Stryker frame, it cannot accommodate other forms of traction. It should never be used for patients with unstable cervical fractures, because when it is turned the pressure on the cervical spine increases as the patient is moved into a "standing" position. Complications associated with the Circ-O-Lectric bed include decubitus ulcers on all bony prominences; therefore use of this bed has decreased dramatically.

Advances in technology have led to the development of many "high-tech" specialty beds. The nurse caring for a patient with multiple orthopaedic injuries must know that not all therapeutic beds can accommodate traction. In concert with the physician you must assess the patient and be familiar with the various beds so the correct bed can be chosen.

One bed often used for patients in traction is the RotoRest Kinetic Treatment Table (KTT) developed by Kinetic Concepts, Inc. The KTT can accommodate balanced suspension skeletal traction as well as cervical traction. It has a unique design that uses a low-profile center-mounted system to transfer the traction forces through flexion cables that absorb the table's motion, allowing the traction to remain stationary throughout the turn.

Advantages of the KTT include maintenance of proper body alignment, decreased risk of contractures, stabilization of long bone fractures throughout rotation, reduction of calcium loss by allowing for the shift in weight-

bearing areas during the turn, and removable parts that allow easy access to the patient for nursing care.

Care of the Patient in a KTT

The KTT can be frightening to both patient and nurse. When you use it for the first time, a company representative can provide inservice education to help decrease the anxiety for all involved.

Place the patient in the center of the bed and adjust and balance the bed before applying traction. The manufacturer's manual describes the appropriate application of traction apparatus. When traction is applied, replace all pads before operating the bed. If the traction is bulky and one sided, use sandbags to provide equal weight on the opposite side for counterbalance.

Because the table rotates at least 20 out of 24 hours per day, check the patient's environment. Position extraneous equipment so it does not interfere with the table's rotation. Secure the safety straps across the patient at all times and place all adjustable bed knobs in the locked position before initiating turning. Tape all tubes and lines (IVs, A-lines, etc.) at their junctions and drape them off the bed. If the patient is respirator dependent, position the respirator with enough tubing to accommodate the bed's rotation and prevent tracheal irritation.

Observe the placement of the tubes and lines through at least one complete rotation to ensure that there is enough room for unobstructed movement, to see that the tubes are not stretched, and to ascertain that the patient is—and feels—secure. The KTT rotates slowly enough that most treatments can be accomplished while the patient is in motion. If this is not feasible, the bed can be stopped for up to 30 minutes.

RELATED NURSING DIAGNOSES

Alteration in Skin Integrity: Related to bedrest, traction, immobility, and motion of the KTT

Assessment	Rationale
Assess all bony prominences	Skin breakdown can occur during treatment on KTT because of shearing forces caused by patient's sliding on mattress
Assess for pressure from removable parts of bed	Proper placement of removable parts decreases risk of abnormal pressure areas
Assess patient's complaints of pain	May indicate area of concern not evident on initial examination (e.g., deep bruise)
Assess neurovascular status	Early recognition of neurovascular impairment helps to decrease risk of long-term, possibly permanent, sequelae
Assess for swelling of extremity(ies)	May indicate compartment syndrome
Assess nutritional status and hydration	A malnourished (depleted protein stores) or dehydrated patient is at increased risk of skin breakdown
Assess patient's mental status	A confused or agitated patient may be more prone to skin breakdown with excessive movement; also more prone to incontinence and noncompliance

Interventions

1. Make sure that all removable parts are secure so turning does not cause irritation.
2. Allow the back and buttocks to be exposed to the air at least once every 4 hours by removing those portions of the bed. Perform skin care at these times.
3. Make sure that the patient's skin remains clean and dry.
4. Remove foot pads at least every 2 hours to avoid irritating the soles and to allow for exercise. (See Chapter 9.)
5. Monitor for irritation about the ears.
6. Adjust head packs as needed and reverse them if called for. (Refer to the manufacturer's manual for specific directions.)
7. Provide nutritional supplements for a patient who cannot eat or has difficulty eating.

Pain: Related to injury and motion of the KTT

Assessment	Rationale
Assess for signs and symptoms of pain	Traction may need to be adjusted, or analgesia may be ineffective
Assess patient's reaction to KTT motion	If patient becomes "seasick," will need antiemetic medication

Interventions

1. Provide analgesics as ordered.
2. Encourage alternative methods of pain control if appropriate.
3. Provide antiemetic medications if the patient becomes nauseated from motion of the bed.
4. To decrease the effects of constant motion, instruct the patient to focus on one object.

Ineffective Coping: Related to injury

Assessment	Rationale
Assess patient's decreased ability to perform self-care activities or any other change in emotional response	Disinterest in personal hygiene may indicate depression or withdrawal
Evaluate patient's support system	Support from family and friends maintains self-esteem and motivates patient to get well

Interventions

1. Allow the patient to verbalize feelings, making sure to stand where you can be seen.

2. Use touch to provide comfort and security.

3. Provide methods of distraction (e.g., a radio or TV) if possible.

4. Hang a large mirror so the patient can see the surroundings and maintain orientation.

5. Provide a large calendar and a few personal belongings (pictures of loved ones, a special stuffed animal) to facilitate orientation.

6. Organize care so the patient is allowed periods of uninterrupted sleep.

Self-care Deficits: Related to the injury and position in bed

Assessment	Rationale
Assess for ability to perform ADLs	Patient may need help in providing basic needs or adapting to situation
Assess for ability to maintain bowel control	KTT may stimulate peristalsis, causing diarrhea, which increases risk of skin breakdown and lowers patient's self-esteem

Interventions

1. Provide all aspects of nursing care as necessary.

2. Encourage the patient to do as much as possible. This facilitates moving the upper extremities and boosts self-esteem.

3. Monitor intake and output. Patients treated on oscillating beds may develop diarrhea due to the stimulation of peristalsis. If this occurs, institute appropriate treatment modalities such as antidiarrheal medications, meticulous skin care, and diet modifications.

Alteration in Gas Exchange: Related to position and injury

Assessment	Rationale
Assess patient for decreased breath sounds, rales or rhonchi, and wheezing	May indicate compromised respiratory status (e.g., hypostatic pneumonia)
Assess vital signs, including temperature, pulse, and respirations	Alterations may indicate impaired gas exchange; early intervention is possible

Interventions

1. Encourage the patient to cough and deep-breathe every 2 to 4 hours.

2. Encourage the use of incentive spirometry.

3. Perform suctioning while the patient is in the extreme right or left lateral positions. The bed does not have to be stopped during the suctioning procedure.

▼

CARE GUIDE
BOEHLER-BRAUN FRAME

The following information should be used in conjunction with the information found in the general traction management guide (Chapter 3).

MECHANICAL COMPONENTS

1. Weights . . . .
   - a. Prescribed amount by physician
   - b. Secure
   - c. Hanging freely
     - (1) Not caught on bed
     - (2) Not resting on floor

2. Pulleys . . . .
   - a. Integral part of frame
   - b. Wheels move freely

3. Ropes . . . .
   - a. In groove of pulley
   - b. No fraying
   - c. Knots securely tied and taped to prevent slipping

4. Countertraction . . . .
   - a. Countertraction provided by the thigh resting against the inclined plane of the frame

5. Bed . . . .
   - a. Firm mattress
   - b. Side rails
   - c. Bed boards (if applicable)

6. Trapeze . . . .
   - a. See general traction management guide (Chapter 3)

PATIENT ALIGNMENT

1. Traction pull . . . .
   - a. Traction is effective, not resting against frame
   - b. Patient is straight in bed with buttocks positioned at break of mattress

     c. Thigh is resting against inclined plane of frame

     d. Head of bed elevated no more than 35 degrees

2. Leg in Boehler-Braun frame . . . .

     a. Should be straight

     b. Slings are clean and equally taut

     c. Slings adequate in number to give even support to extremity

     d. Slings placed so there is no pressure on popliteal space, Achilles tendon, or heel

     e. Proximal end of frame should not press into perineum; protect with sheepskin padding

3. Provision of comfort when moving patient . .

     a. Explain procedure to patient

     b. Teach patient to use trapeze

     c. Teach patient to use siderail to help in turning

     d. Use firm and steady motion, avoiding bumping or jarring frame

     e. Sheets are applied in manner that eliminates need to move frame at each bed change

     f. **Get help when needed**

     g. When moving patient from bed to stretcher (at least 2 people guiding and supporting frame and 2 people helping patient)

     h. **Do not interrupt traction when moving patient—guide, but do not lift, weights**

NURSING CARE

1. Maintenance of skin integrity . . . .

     a. Check pressure points

       (1) See general traction management guide (Chapter 3)

       (2) Check groin, perineum, and genitalia

       (3) Lower extremity: Achilles tendon, heel, popliteal area, head of fibula

b. Check for increased risk of skin breakdown
   (1) See general traction management guide
       (Chapter 3)
c. Adjunct equipment to decrease risk
   (1) See general traction management guide
       (Chapter 3)

2. Alteration in tissue perfusion . . . .   a. See general traction management guide
   (Chapter 3)

3. Potential for pin site infection . . . .   a. Check pin sites for redness, warmth, edema,
   pain, prolonged drainage
   b. Check to see that pin site is clean and free
      of encrustations
   c. Check for migration of pin
   d. Check that patient is receiving prescribed
      pin site care
   e. Instruct patient not to touch around pin site

4. Alteration in neurological status . . . .   a. See general traction management guide
   (Chapter 3)

5. Alteration in gas exchange . . . .   a. See general traction management guide
   Chapter 3)

6. Alteration in nutritional status . . . .   a. See general traction management guide
   (Chapter 3)

7. Alteration in elimination . . . .   a. See general traction management guide
   (Chapter 3)

8. Impaired physical mobility . . . .   a. See general traction guide (Chapter 3)

9. Ineffective coping . . . .   a. See general traction management guide
   (Chapter 3)

Discharge Planning for Patients in Traction

Both cost-containment measures and the advances in home care services are responsible for patients' being discharged to home with a continued need for traction. Patients are assessed for the level of care needed and allowed to go home as soon as they no longer require hospital-level care. Those remaining in hospital need frequent medical attention and intervention and/or 24-hour skilled nursing care. When the patient is medically stable, when adjustments have been made in the traction application, and when 24-hour nursing care is no longer needed, a discharge plan is instituted. The plan includes intermittent nursing visits, intermittent physical therapy visits, and visits by a home health aide for personal care.

The patient going home in traction usually needs a family member or other person who is willing, available, and able to learn how to care for the patient. This person must also understand the traction application and be able to provide all custodial care.

Examples of patients who can be cared for at home are infants needing divarication traction, patients needing several weeks of balanced-suspension traction, and individuals with external fixation devices in place.

Discharge Planning for Patients in Traction

Discharge planning is an integral part of the continuity of care. Continuity of care is an interdisciplinary process that involves patients and their families, requires development of a plan, facilitates the patient's transition from one care setting to another, and is based on the patient's changing needs and available resources. The discharge planning process identifies the needs of the patient, assesses the resources to meet those needs, and provides the patient with the most appropriate level of care. The goal of discharge planning is the smooth transition of a patient from one level of care to another.

Who Does Discharge Planning?

All health professionals providing care to a patient are involved in discharge planning to varying degrees. In this dynamic process all concerned persons provide input, beginning at admission, through care provision, and until the patient is discharged. Persons concerned with discharge planning include hospital-based staff, community-based staff, the patient, and the patient's family.

Discharge planning services for patients vary from hospital to hospital. Sometimes a discharge planning coordinator carries out the total process; sometimes the coordinator provides services only for patients with complex needs.

When caring for a patient in traction, you must understand the steps in the discharge planning process and be able to carry out appropriate planning functions.

How the Discharge-Planning Process is Integrated into the Nursing Process for Patients in Traction

The steps in discharge planning are an integral part of the nursing process and can be summarized as follows:

1. Screening
2. Assessment
3. Planning
4. Implementation
5. Evaluation

Screening

In this step you identify the patient with discharge problems. All patients who are in traction have discharge needs, but not all have problems. At a minimum, you must screen all patients for risk factors related to their orthopaedic problem and other medical conditions. In children and the elderly, traction is usually only one of the problems to be addressed when considering discharge needs.

Assessment

In this step you determine the patient's needs and the resources to meet those needs. This complex process forms the basis on which other steps may depend. It includes identifying the patient's current and future physical and psychosocial needs, the support systems available, and the location to which the patient will be discharged. It requires collaboration with the physician, therapists, social workers, and other health professionals who may be involved in the delivery of care for the patient in traction or following the removal of traction.

In assessing the discharge needs for a patient in traction, you must consider needs other than those related to the traction. Some of these are wound care, nutrition, pain management, and monitoring of cardiopulmonary status.

Planning

An initial plan is made after all problems are identified and is modified as the patient progresses through the course of care. The plan for discharge is based on the assessed patient needs at discharge. Decisions must be made by all parties involved, especially the physician, patient, and family, about the plan for ongoing care.

Implementation

Implementation includes making referrals to other care providers, agencies, or companies; arranging for patient and family education; securing needed health care resources; completing necessary referral forms; and making follow-up appointments. The plan of care is directly related to the length of time the patient must be in traction, the patient's weight-bearing status, and the availability of a support system.

Evaluation

Evaluation of the discharge planning process is done on an ongoing basis. Changes are made as new information is gathered and as a more definite plan is identified. The plan changes as the patient progresses in ambulation and self-care and as the family can demonstrate capability in providing care.

NURSING DIAGNOSES AND THE IMPACT THESE HAVE ON THE DISCHARGE PLANNING PROCESS FOR PATIENTS IN TRACTION

Activity Intolerance Related to Restrictions of the Traction Apparatus and Physical Injury

1. Alteration in ambulatory status: When discharging a patient in traction, you must assess the degree of interruption in the patient's ambulatory status. If the patient will be in traction 24 hours a day, confined to bed, or limited in the amount of time out of bed, make a referral to the discharge planning coordinator (if one is available) for assistance in carrying out a full evaluation. This patient will need assistance with personal care and with preparing and eating food. He or she must also be monitored for skin integrity, bowel and bladder function, and other problems associated with immobility. Even though the patient will be cared for at home, the potential problems related to immobility still exist; teaching the patient and caregiver about these is essential.

2. Alteration in weight-bearing status related to the type of injury: If the patient can be out of traction for a limited time but is partial or non–weight bearing, consult with a physical therapist to determine the safest method of ambulation. If the patient's mobility is limited, assess the home environment to determine the need for ramps, railings, or other safety considerations. The proximity of bedroom to bathroom and kitchen and the number of stairs between living areas bear on the need for equipment. If the patient will be ambulatory at home, refer to a home physical therapist.

Another consideration is whether the patient can get in and out of the traction alone. If the traction apparatus must be assembled and reattached, you must teach this procedure before discharge.

3. Alteration in mobility related to the inability to sit for a prolonged time: Patients in vertebral traction must be either lying or standing; they cannot sit for long periods. Their initial problem involves getting home. If they live a great distance from the hospital and the length of time for the trip exceeds the time permitted for sitting, an ambulance may be needed. Modify the schedule of care to meet this activity restriction; for example, meals with the family should coincide with the times the patient is allowed to sit. Skin care to the shoulders, head, coccyx, heels, and elbows is important to relieve the constant pressure caused by being in a supine position.

Self-care Deficit Related to the Traction Application

1. The number of extremities involved in the traction or functionally is important. For example, a patient in skeletal traction for the lower extremity, with a fractured arm, will need additional assistance.

2. The weight-bearing status of the patient directly affects self-care. Patients who are non–weight bearing in the lower extremities may still carry out some self-care, such as washing, grooming, and eating. If they are non–weight bearing in the upper extremities, more compromise of function is present. They may not be able to use a transfer board, connect a traction apparatus, or even eat indepen-

dently. Arm involvement is sometimes more complicated from a self-care point of view than involvement of one or both legs.

Skin Integrity and Potential Impairment Caused by Traction Application to the Skin and Prolonged Bedrest

1. The patient at home in traction risks skin breakdown because of the traction apparatus and prolonged bedrest. Also the patient cannot observe all potential problem areas. An individual in a head halter, for example, cannot easily look at the back of the head, shoulders, or coccyx. Teach the patient to use a mirror to view these areas and to be aware of the symptoms of possible skin breakdown (e.g., tingling, numbness, soft spots, or other seemingly minor discomforts). These are usually the first signs of problems and must be addressed as soon as possible. The patient's caregiver must be taught to observe for potential skin problems.

2. If the patient is being discharged in skeletal traction, teach both the patient and the caregiver how to care for the pin sites. This will include how to clean the pin site and what specific observations to make. (See Chapter 6.)

Pain and Discomfort Related to Traction Application and Posttrauma Effects

By the time the patient is discharged in traction, pain usually is not a problem. The patient should be stable, relatively pain free, or on a pain-control regimen before being discharged.

Teach the patient and caregiver to contact the physician if pain develops or changes, since this indicates a possible problem with the traction, or another medical condition that may need evaluation.

Comfort measures such as positioning, massage, or diversional therapy may be helpful.

Constipation Related to Change in Intake and Prolonged Bedrest; Potential for Bladder Distention Related to Delayed Emptying of Bladder

When the patient is stable, seek to reestablish the elimination pattern that existed before injury or surgery. Prolonged bedrest in traction may impact on bowel function. Establish a routine as close to normal as possible. The patient may need a bedpan or bedside commode if confined to bed or when allowed out of traction for only short periods. A fracture pan may also help. These items allow the patient to void and defecate when needed and may prevent incontinence, overdistention of the bladder, or constipation.

Role Performance Altered Because of Changed Ability to Resume a Role

The degree of role interruption for a patient being discharged in traction depends on the type of traction, the patient's ambulatory status, and the level of dependence for self-care. You must assess functional needs to ascertain what referrals the patient will need. For example, if the patient's employment will be interrupted for more time than allowed by sick benefits, if child care is needed, if an elderly person is being cared for, or if schooling will be interrupted, the patient is likely to benefit from a social service referral.

Role reversal is a problem when the person who has been the caregiver suddenly becomes the person needing care. In this situation, working through psychosocial problems must begin before care is taught.

Knowledge Deficit Related to Postacute Care

Depending on the type of traction and the overall status of the patient, you must provide teaching to meet all the patient's needs. Factors influencing the teaching plan will revolve around the patient's destination and the complexity of the care needed. For example, a patient being discharged to another facility to receive care will not need as extensive teaching as a patient who is going home.

For patients who are going home, review the following topics as soon as the patient is medically and psychologically ready for teaching:

1. Traction apparatus set-up and mechanical components. Teach the patient to observe the traction apparatus with the same degree of thoroughness as you have been doing in the hospital. For example, the patient must be able to watch for frayed ropes, loose knots, or other mechanical components of the traction set-up.
2. If the patient is being discharged with an external fixator or skeletal traction, instruct him or her in the procedure for pin site care.
3. Teach skin care, including what to look for, how to wash and dry the skin, what lotions to use, how to prevent irritation from the traction apparatus, how to move in bed to prevent skin irritation, and the importance of adequate nutrition and fluids.
4. Demonstrate how to make an occupied bed. To maintain the traction and avoid skin trauma, the bed linen for a traction patient must be replaced carefully.
5. Review the signs and symptoms of potential complications: specifically, impaired respiratory status, neurovascular symp-

toms (need immediate attention), signs of phlebitis, and dehydration. Instruct the patient to take his or her temperature every day; inspect the pin site for redness, drainage, "tenting," or slippage; observe the affected extremity for signs of neurological compromise, including numbness, tingling, or the inability to move; and check the circulation on a regular basis. Instruct the patient in how to take a pulse, blanch the skin, and compare the color or warmth of an extremity. Be sure to emphasize that pain in the calf, especially pain that increases when the toes are pointed toward the head, must be reported to the physician **immediately,** as should any sudden onset of chest pain, feeling of pressure in the chest, or shortness of breath.

When teaching the patient or significant other in preparation for discharge, assess that person's ability to comprehend your instruction. Knowing that the patient is anxious about the discharge, that many things must be learned in a short time, and that it is important to make critical observations, you may recommend to the discharge planning coordinator that a referral be made for a home care nurse to continue, reinforce, or validate teaching.

Types of Postacute Care Services Available for the Patient in Traction

Postacute care services include transfer to another hospital, transfer to a rehabilitation facility, transfer to a nursing facility, discharge to home with services, and discharge to home without services. Those participating in the decision about the patient's destination are the physician, therapist (both physical and occupational), primary nurse, and patient and family.

Often a case manager is assigned by the patient's insurance company. This individual will become involved in discharge planning by determining resources covered by the insurer and by negotiating for services the patient needs.

The patient's level of care need determines where he or she will receive the best possible postacute care. These general statements apply to postacute options for the patient in traction:

1. Transfer to another acute care setting: Usually done when the patient is medically unstable and needs the level of care of a tertiary-care hospital. Decision made by physicians at the referring and receiving hospitals.

2. Transfer to a rehabilitation facility: Done when the patient (a) is no longer in need of hospital-level care but is not yet independent enough to be discharged to home care or (b) would benefit from the intensity of therapy at a rehabilitation facility. Usually patients in traction are not discharged to a rehabilitation facility because they would not be able to tolerate the intensity of therapy.

3. Transfer to a nursing facility: Done when the patient has skilled care needs that cannot be met at home. This patient usually requires 24-hour monitoring, needs the assistance of more than one person to get out of bed (if he is able to), and has multiple deficits in activities of daily living (ADLs). The family or caregiver may not be able to provide the level of care the patient needs.

4. Discharge to home with services: Done when the patient with extensive needs has an adequate support structure. Services available in the home include nursing, physical and occupational therapy, health aides, and social services. Equipment for traction is available, as are patient education on its use and maintenance services.

5. Discharge to home without services: Done if the patient is totally independent in self-care activities and has shown proficiency in setting up and taking down the traction and in observing all skin surfaces that will be contacting the traction apparatus. This patient must not be home bound but must be able to get to the physician's office for medical follow-up.

Traction in the Home Setting

The discharge-planning process carried out by the nurse in the acute-care setting will make it easier for the patient to be released to his or her home. The assessment of patient needs and the resources to meet those needs should be made as soon as it is determined that the patient is going home in traction and will be done in the context of all other identified needs of the patient as they relate to (1) the application of traction and (2) the functional dependence on traction. A patient in traction at home frequently has other medical conditions that must be addressed (e.g., cardiovascular monitoring and wound care), especially if he has a traumatic injury. This chapter addresses these as well.

The physician, nurse, and physical therapist should collaborate in assessing the needs of the patient and the potential needs of care at home. The services available to the patient at home include skilled services (e.g., nursing, physical and occupational therapy), social services, and dietary services as well as visits by a home health aide. Other community-based services include home-delivered meals, housecleaning, and the performance of errands and chores.

Assessment of the patient should be done as close to the time of discharge as possible so the patient's ability to manage self-care can be accurately evaluated.

The following areas of patient need should be assessed and the findings incorporated into the plan for home care.

- How will the patient manage the activities of daily living, such as eating, toileting, bathing, dressing, and, if allowed, transferring from bed to chair or bed to standing position?
- How will the patient's change in activity affect his nutritional and metabolic needs?
- Will the patient be able to perform range of motion exercises to the unaffected extremities?
- How will the patient and family adjust to continued needs and interruption in their usual life-style?
- Are there other patient needs related to health issues such as diabetes, cardiovascular disease, or traumatic injuries?
- Will the patient need ongoing laboratory tests, such as those for managing anticoagulant therapy?
- How will the patient get to the physician's office for follow-up care?
- Do the patient and significant other understand the signs and symptoms of potential complications related to traction application?
- Is there a family member or significant other who can provide the necessary care for the patient in the home? How much

assistance does the family need for personal care, meals, and monitoring the patient's progress?

- Does the patient have a skilled care need that can be met only by a licensed practitioner (e.g., skeletal traction set-up, a pin site that needs care, skin breakdown, or a change in metabolic or cardiovascular status)?
- Does the patient have medical insurance that will help pay for needed services? Has the insurance company been contacted to determine whether home care services are covered?
- Is the patient's home environment conducive to recovery (i.e., easy access into and out of the house, bathroom convenient to the patient, phone for emergency use)?
- Will the patient need a special bed for the application of traction, and does it fit in the patient's home?
- Does the patient know how to do pin site care and are there supplies for the procedure?
- Will the patient be able to resume the instrumental activities of daily living (IADLs), such as telephoning and managing money affairs?

After the needs of the patient are identified and it is determined that the patient can be cared for at home, a referral should be made to a licensed home care agency that can provide for these needs. The nurse should seek assistance from the hospital-based discharge planner to help the patient and family select an appropriate agency.

The physician must be involved in the discharge plans specifically in writing discharge orders for the home care agency to follow.

Nursing Interventions

When the patient is admitted to service by a home care agency you must establish an individualized plan of care to address the following points:

1. The patient's diagnosis, including the reason for traction
2. The rehabilitation potential and short- and long-term goals
3. The patient's needs and any potential problems in meeting those needs
4. Problems associated with the family support system
5. Types and frequency of services to be provided, including medication administration, nutrition needs, procedures, equipment, and transportation
6. Functional limitations of the patient, particularly regarding ambulation
7. Safety measures to protect the patient from complications and additional injury
8. Psychosocial needs of the patient, especially those related to the interruption of work, school, or other social activities
9. Patient and family education

The initiation of the home care plan is done by the home care nurse and is established within the time frames requested by the referring physician. The patient should be visited within 24 hours of discharge from the hospital.

Your care plan should include the following points:

- Observing the patient and family in skin care, equipment safety, pin site care, nutrition planning, fluid and electrolyte balance, signs of complications and the need for follow-up medical care, and medication compliance
- Monitoring skin care
- Monitoring bowel and bladder function

- Assisting in obtaining laboratory studies for the patient who is on anticoagulant therapy
- Observing ROM exercises for all joints
- Assessing the patient for symptoms of other diseases or the exacerbation of existing diseases
- Assisting the patient and family with stress and coping strategies
- Coordinating all care being rendered to the patient, including that provided by the orthopaedic surgeon, other physicians (surgeons, cardiologists, endocrinologists, other health professionals), and the family or significant others

Physical Therapy Services

A referral to a physical therapist is required at discharge in the following situations:

1. The patient has loss of function of an extremity and will need restorative care.
2. There is an exacerbation of a chronic disease causing decreased physical functioning.
3. The patient needs special physical therapy modalities such as ultrasound or neurostimulation.
4. The patient's weight is such that special techniques are needed to allow the patient to move in bed and to permit the home health aide or family to perform adequate skin care, provide a bedpan, or change the bed linen.
5. The patient needs instruction on techniques to restore strength or increase strength in preparation for future ambulation.

Before traction is discontinued in the home, the physician should request the services of a physical therapist. The physical therapist will visit the patient prior to the discontinuation of the traction to do the following:

1. Assess the safety of the home environment in relation to such things as removal of rugs, installation of safety hand rails, or construction of ramps.
2. Assess the type of assistive devices needed for transfer from the bed and for progressive ambulation. The patient may need things like a transfer board, a wheelchair with removable arms and leg elevators, or a walker, crutches, or cane.
3. Evaluate the need for a commode early in ambulation, since the patient may not be strong enough to walk long distances to the bathroom, or the bathroom may not accommodate a wheelchair or walker.
4. Evaluate the patient's balance and coordination and make recommendations on activities to improve them in anticipation of ambulation.

When the traction is discontinued a physical therapist should do the following:

1. Evaluate the range of motion of the affected extremity
2. Institute ROM exercises
3. Begin transfer techniques
4. Assess the patient's strength and balance and make recommendations for the patient, family, and home health aide on techniques for improvement

Occupational Therapy Services

The services of an occupational therapist can also be utilized for the patient who has traction in the home setting. An occupational therapist is best utilized when the patient

- Needs evaluation of motor skills and strength of the upper extremities

- Needs assessment of joint inflammation and pain with instruction in joint protection techniques, pain management skills, and supportive devices such as splints or slings.
- Needs assessment of cognitive and perceptual motor abilities while in traction.

Nutritionist or Dietitian Services

The services of a nutritionist or dietitian may be requested for patients with the following problems:

1. Obesity (The patient will be immobilized and thus require fewer calories, and no adjustment in caloric intake or quality could cause a gain in weight.)
2. Diabetes or a cardiovascular problem requiring assessment and management
3. Decreased functional ability, particularly related to eating in a supine position (Recommendations may include changes in the presentation of foods [finger foods] or a soft or semisoft diet. Patients with activity changes also frequently become constipated and require a change in diet to prevent this problem. Fluid intake strategies, if appropriate for the patient, may be implemented.)
4. Cultural or ethnic dietary diversity (For example, the patient may need to learn the caloric content of some foods prepared by the family.)

Social Services

A referral for social services may be appropriate for patients in traction who have experienced trauma and its associated problems, for those who will be out of work or school for pro-longed periods, or for those who may experience prolonged disability as a result of their condition.

Home Health Aide Services

A home health aide works under the direction and supervision of a registered nurse who works for a home health agency. Home health aide services should be requested for patients who will need personal care assistance in tasks such as bathing, toileting, and eating and some environmental tasks such as changing bed linen and doing light housework.

A home health aide provides essential assistance to the patient and respite for family members. Respite care is defined as the care provided for a patient that normally could be provided by a family member but cannot be done on a 24-hour 7-day-a-week basis.

Home Medical Equipment Supplies and Services for Traction

Traction in the home must be coordinated with both a home nursing agency and a home medical equipment company. These companies have specialized equipment for the home and also provide servicing of equipment and patient and family education in the use of the equipment.

Traction equipment for use in the home is ordered before the patient is discharged from the hospital. The equipment must be delivered and set up so there will be no interruption in the traction.

The type of traction determines the equipment needed. For example, balanced-suspension traction will require a hospital bed with a traction frame that can support the traction appliances, a trapeze, side rails, and blocks to put under the bed for countertraction. A variety of 1-, 2-, and 5-pound weights should also be ordered. They can be used in combination to provide the prescribed amount of traction and countertraction. For example, 6 pounds of weight can be accomplished using a 5-pound and a 1-pound weight, or three 2-pound weights. Sometimes, bags filled with water to specified levels are used in traction applications.

Since the set-up at home should be similar to that in the hospital, the equipment company representative will visit the patient in the hospital to do a full inventory of the type and amount of equipment needed—itemizing pulleys, ropes, spreader bars, suspension equipment, hospital bed type, traction frame, skin protection mattress cover, side rails, elevating blocks, and trapeze. A traction set-up can be compromised if even one pulley is missing.

Several purchases by the family are recommended:

1. Sheets for the bed so regular linen changes can be made
2. Pillows with covers for positioning the patient
3. Bed pads, commonly called "incontinence pads"; these should be used carefully because they wrinkle easily and can be a source of discomfort to the patient, even compromising skin integrity if ridges are allowed to develop and persist under the patient; although they are recommended for incontinent patients, the family should be instructed to inspect them frequently and check the patient's skin for irritation
4. An overbed table and portable phone; these will allow the patient more independence and lessen the danger that the trac-

tion is interrupted or a joint is injured while trying to reach for items
5. A call bell to be used by the patient to signal for assistance

Transportation for the Patient from Hospital to Home

Transportation home should take into account the time the patient is allowed out of traction. If traction cannot be interrupted for the trip home, an ambulance may be needed. Consult the physician for precautionary steps that may be needed in transferring the patient from the hospital bed to the stretcher to the bed at home.

Occasionally a traction frame or other portable traction application can be used to transport the patient, but this must be arranged in advance. If it is allowed, the nurse, therapist, or a specially trained orthopaedic technician must accompany the patient throughout the transfer process and assist in reestablishing the traction set-up in the home.

The "windmill transfer traction" uses an existing skeletal pin to maintain traction during transfer. It is based on the windlass method used by Army field hospitals. This method continues the proper distraction of a fracture while providing desired knee and hip flexion. Wraps above and below the pin site prevent adverse rotation of the extremity. When this method is used to wrap the extremity, the Thomas splint is disconnected from suspension and the patient can be transported. At home the extremity is placed back in balanced suspension and the windlass transfer system is removed. When the patient has been safely placed in traction, it is advisable to take pictures of the traction application for future reference.

Community Safety Concerns

Whenever a patient is confined to home and would need extraordinary assistance in evacuating the building in the event of fire or other disaster, the local police and fire departments should be notified before the patient is discharged from the hospital as to where in the home the patient will be located.

Financial Considerations of Home Care

Most insurers, including Medicare, provide some level of home care service for patients in traction. Restrictions vary from one insurer to another. For example, for home care services to be covered by Medicare, they must be ordered by a physician, the patient must be confined to the home (i.e., unable to leave without assistance), the care must be intermittent (not requiring 24 hours of skilled nursing care), and the patient must need the level of care termed "skilled" (i.e., the services of a licensed nurse or therapist). If the patient needs only the services of a home health aide, he or she must pay privately for the services.

To minimize the potential financial liability of patients receiving care, you must investigate all available payment sources and obtain prior authorization whenever possible. Care for the patient in the home is usually cost effective when compared to hospital care, but adding ancillary services such as home health aides or multiple professional services can make cost a significant factor in deciding to move the patient home. The prudent use of all resources, including health professionals, family, significant others, and volunteers, can greatly impact the cost of therapy and may provide a feeling of self-confidence for the patient and family support network.

Specific Traction Applications and Determining a Plan of Care

To assess the different types of traction correctly, refer to the chapter that discusses the application desired. The information found there can offer guidelines in establishing a plan of care, planning for patient teaching, and setting up a system of observations for monitoring the signs and symptoms suggestive of complications.

Glossary

A

Abduct: To move away from the midline of the body

Acetabulum: Socket in the hip bone (innominate bone, i.e., the ilium, ischium, and pubis) into which the head of the femur fits

Achilles tendon: Strong band of tissue at the back of the heel that connects the calf muscles to the heel bone (calcaneus)

Activities of daily living (ADLs): All activities that permit a person to function independently in daily life; the term refers to personal care (hygiene, dressing), homemaking, and ambulation

Adduct: To move toward the midline of the body

Agitation: Disturbed and excited state

Alignment: Keeping the part of the body in traction in line with the pull of the weight

Alveolocapillaries: Thin-walled structures of the lungs surrounded by networks of capillaries, through whose walls the exchange of carbon dioxide and oxygen takes place

Angulation: Formation of angles

Ankle circling: Moving the foot in a circle through the full range of ankle motion

Anterior: Before or in front of

Anterolateral: In front of and on the outer side

Aspiration: To withdraw fluid by negative pressure or suction

Atrophy: Wasting with a decrease in size of a normally developed tissue or organ; may be due to disuse, disease, lack of nutrition, or injury to the nerves

Axis: Straight line through the center of the body or a bone.

B

Babinski reflex: Dorsiflexion of the big toe with extension and fanning of the other toes elicited by firmly stroking the lateral aspect of the sole of the foot; it is a normal reaction in infants but abnormal in children and adults, indicating a lesion in the pyramidal tract

Blanching sign: Circulation check, by which pressure is applied to the skin or nailbed with the finger and then quickly released; the return of blood to the capillaries (capillary filling) is demonstrated

Blood gases (arterial blood gases, ABGs): Measurement of the arterial acid-base balance, PO_2, PCO_2, and bicarbonate (HCO_3^-) concentrations, used in assessing a patient's respiratory and metabolic state

C

Callus: Bonelike material produced during healing between the ends of a fractured bone

Calcaneus: Heel bone (os calcis)

Calculi: Small hard masses (stones) formed in hollow organs of the body or their passages.

Cervical: Pertaining to the neck; the first seven vertebrae of the spinal column are the cervical vertebrae

Circumduction: Circular movement of a limb

Circumferential: Referring to a line that bounds a circle or spherical body or goes around a body part.

Coccygeal: Pertaining to the coccyx

Coccyx: Last four bones of the spine; usually fused and articulating with the sacrum

Comminuted: Describing a fracture in which the bone is broken into more than two segments

Compartment syndrome: Progressive condition or series of symptoms that results from interference of blood flow to part of an extremity; a cycle of edema and ischemia that, if unchecked, will result in a deformed and nonfunctioning limb

Compound (open) fracture: See under Fracture

Compression: Act of pressing upon or together; the state of being pressed together, as in compression dressing

Condyles: Rounded portions (two) at the ends of a bone

Conjunctiva: Membrane lining the inner surface of the eyelids and covering the eyeball

Contraction: Shortening of a muscle or reduction in its size

Contractures: Abnormal shortening of muscle tissue, makes the muscle highly resistant to stretching but can lead to permanent disability

Convulsion: Violent and involuntary spasm or contraction of a group of muscles

Congenital: Present and existing at the time of birth

Congenital hip (CDH): Usually refers to congenital dislocation of the hip; most common of the congenital disorders, in which the femoral head may be subluxed or completely dislocated out of the acetabulum

Countertraction: Pull in opposition to the traction force

Cyanosis: Bluish discoloration of the skin and mucous membranes, caused by oxygen deficiency and an excess of carbon dioxide in the blood

D

Debilitation: Weakened condition

Decubitus: Act of lying down

    Lateral decubitus: Lying on one side

    Decubitus ulcer: Ulceration resulting from local interference with circulation (also called bedsore or pressure sore); usually occurs over a bony prominence

Deficit: Less than normal

Delirium tremens: Serious mental state accompanied by hallucinations, extreme restlessness, agitation, and uncontrollable shaking resulting from excessive, chronic use of alcohol

Developmental dysplastic hip (DDH): Abnormal development of the hip joint (see Congenital hip)

Devitalized: Destruction or loss of viability as in devitalized tissue or bone

Diaphragmatic: Pertaining to the diaphragm

Dislocation: When two bones that make up a joint are completely separated and no longer articulate

Distal: Area farthest from a point of reference or the point of attachment or origin

Divarication traction: Used in hip dislocations in children to produce a gradual or progressive reduction of a dislocation; accomplished by use of Bryant traction

Dorsiflexion: Act of bending a part backward (e.g., flexing the ankle so the toes are directed toward the knee)

Dorsum: Posterior or superior surface of a body or body part, as of the foot or hand

Dysplastic: Abnormal development of a tissue (e.g., bone)

Dyspnea: Difficult or labored breathing

E

Edema: Abnormal accumulation of fluid in the tissues

Edentulous: Without teeth

Embolus: Mass of undissolved material, usually part or all of a thrombus, carried in the bloodstream and frequently causing obstruction of a vessel

Equinovarus: Angulation of the foot downward and toward the midline of the body

Exercise: Performance of physical activity for purposes of conditioning the body, improving health, maintaining fitness, correcting a deformity, or restoring the organs and bodily functions to a state of health; any action, skill, or maneuver that exerts the muscles and is performed repeatedly to develop or strengthen the body or any of its parts

  Active: When the patient uses his own muscles to do the exercise

  Passive: When the patient does not use his own muscles independently; these exercises must be done to the patient by another person or with the help of an assistive device

Extension: Straightening of the joint (extremity)

External rotation: Outward turning of an extremity

Exudate: Material that has escaped from blood vessels and accumulated in tissues or on tissue surfaces, usually as a result of inflammation

F

Fat embolism syndrome (FES): Progression of a series of symptoms caused by release of fat droplets into the bloodstream.

Fascia: Strong sheet of connective tissue surrounding and connecting muscle

Fasciotomy: Incision (dissection) of a fascia

Femoral neck: Area of the femur between the head and the greater and lesser trochanters

Flexion: Bending of a joint or extremity

Foot drop: Condition in which the patient is unable to dorsiflex the foot

Fracture: Break in the continuity of a bone

  Simple (closed) fracture: An undisplaced fracture

  Compound (open) fracture: When the bone communicates with the outside environment; the skin may be broken from within by bone fragments or from without by an external force

  Comminuted fracture: When the bone is broken in more than two fragments

  Greenstick fracture: When the fracture involves only one cortex of the bone; usually occurs in children

G

Gangrene: Death and putrefaction of body tissue caused by loss of circulation to the area; often results from infection or injury

Girdlestone: Procedure named for Dr. Girdlestone in which the hip joint is removed and the joint space is allowed to fill in with fibrous tissue; the patient is placed in traction postoperatively so shortening of the extremity will be kept to a minimum

Gluteal fold: Junction of the buttock and posterior thigh

Gluteal setting: Tightening of the gluteal muscles; done in a repetitive pattern as part of an exercise program

Graduated: Arranged by successive steps or degrees

Greater trochanter: Process on the femur at the upper end of its lateral surface

H

Hamstrings: Group of muscles located on the posterior aspect of the thigh—biceps femoris, semitendinosis, and semimembranosis—whose function is to extend the thigh

Hematoma: Extravasated blood in a tissue or cavity (may be clotted)

Hematuria: Presence of blood in the urine

Hemoptysis: Coughing or spitting of blood, resulting from bleeding from any part of the respiratory tract

Herniated disc: Protrusion of the nucleus pulposus from the disc between adjoining vertebrae

Hyperextended: Extended beyond the normal range

Hypoesthesia: State of abnormally decreased sensitivity to stimuli

Hypostatic: Settling of sediment or deposits at the bottom of a fluid (e.g., fluid in a lung in hypostatic pneumonia)

Hypovolemia: Abnormally decreased volume of circulating fluid (plasma) in the body

I

Immobilize: To render motionless, fix in place

Impingment (impinging): To strike, knock against, or be caught upon

Infarction: Development of a localized area of ischemic necrosis produced by occlusion of the arteries or veins supplying a part; may

also result from circulatory stasis secondary to venous occlusion

Internal rotation: Inward rotation of an extremity

Intertrochanteric: Area of the femur between the greater and lesser trochanters

Ischemia: Deficiency of blood supply to a part of the body

K

Kirschner wire: Small-gauge stainless steel wire used in balanced-suspension traction and external fixator devices

L

Lateral: Pertaining to the side; away from the midline of the body

Longitudinal: Running lengthwise

Lucidity: Ability to be rational and clear

M

Malleoli: Two rounded processes (lateral and medial) on the ankle joint at the lower end of the fibula (lateral, external) and the tibia (medial, internal)

Malunion: Healing of a fracture in a position that does not allow satisfactory function

Mechanical: Automatic natural process, done as if by machine independent of thought

Medial: Nearest the midline of the body

Metabolic: Pertaining to metabolism, the sum of the processes involved in the buildup and destruction of cell tissues; the chemical cellular changes providing the energy for life's processes and the elimination of waste materials

Migration: Movement from one place or position to another

N

Necrosis: Death of areas of tissue or bone surrounded by healthy parts; usually caused by loss of blood supply or trauma to the area

Neurovascular: Concerning both the nervous and the vascular systems

O

Occlusion: Act of closure or state of being closed; obstruction of the flow of blood through an artery (e.g., of the heart in coronary occlusion)

Olecranon: The bony projection of the ulna at the elbow.

Open fracture: *See under* Fracture

Osteomyelitis: Inflammation of the bone and/or marrow

Oxygenation: Saturation with oxygen

P

Palsy: Temporary or permanent loss of sensation, motion, or control of movement

Parallelogram: Four-sided figure composed of straight lines and having its opposite sides parallel and equal; usually a figure of greater length than breadth

Paresthesia: Abnormal sensation with no obvious cause (e.g., numbness)

Pearson attachment: Device that helps to convert a Thomas or other splint for balanced-suspension traction; it is fastened to the Thomas splint at the knee and allows passive notion of the knee without disturbing the alignment of the fracture

Perfusion: Passage of fluid through the vessels of a specific organ or body part

Periosteum: Highly specialized connective tissue that covers all bones except joint surfaces; the inner layer contains bone-forming cells; the periosteum is necessary for bone growth, nutrition, and repair

Peroneal nerve: Bundle of neural fibers originating in the sciatic nerve and innervating the calf and foot

Perpendicular: Perfectly upright or vertical and at right angle to a given line

Petechiae: Small, pinpoint, nonraised, round, purple-red spots caused by intradermal or submucosal hemorrhages

Plantarflexion: Motion of the foot at the ankle joint directed downward; extending the ankle and pointing the toes

Pneumonitis: Inflammation of the lung tissue

Popliteal space: Posterior surface of the knee

Posterior: In back of; toward the rear or dorsum

Proximal: Area nearest a point of reference or the point of origin or attachment

Purulent: Containing or consisting of pus

Q

Quadriceps: Group of four muscles—rectus femoris, vastus lateralis, vastus medialis, and vastus intermedius—in the anterior thigh that extend the leg

Quad setting: Tightening of the quadriceps muscles; usually done in a repetitive pattern as part of an exercise program for muscle strengthening

R

Rales pronounced (*rahls*): Abnormal respiratory sounds heard on auscultation and indicating a pathological condition of the lungs

Reduction: To restore to a normal position (as the ends of a fractured bone)

Reflex: Automatic response to a stimulus; does not require the intervention of conscious thought

Reverse Trendelenburg: Supine position with the head higher then the feet

Rhonchi: Coarse dry rales in the bronchi heard on auscultation of the lungs

Rotation: Process of turning on an axis (one object upon another) so the angle between the two objects does not change

S

Sequestrum: Piece of dead bone that has become separated from healthy bone during the process of necrosis

Sloughing: Mass of dead tissue in or separating from living tissue

Sprain: Wrenching or twisting of a joint with partial rupture of its ligaments; there may also be damage to associated blood vessels, muscles, tendons, and nerves

Stabilize: To make firm and steady

Stasis: Stoppage of flow (as of blood or other body fluids)

Steinmann pin: Large-diameter stainless steel wire used in skeletal traction and external fixation devices

Strain: Overstretching or overextension of a muscle

Subluxation: Incomplete or partial dislocation

Subtrochanteric: Area on the femur below the trochanters

Supracondylar: Area above a condyle

Syndrome: Combination of symptoms resulting from a single cause or so commonly oc-

curring together as to constitute a distinct clinical picture

T

Tachycardia: Abnormally rapid heart rate, usually taken to be over 100 beats per minute.

Tachypnea: Rapid respirations; quick and shallow breathing

Temporomandibular joint (TMJ): Articulation of the temporal bone and the mandible

Tenting: Stretching of the skin that surrounds and adheres to a pin, creating a tentlike appearance

Thomas splint: Device for stabilizing a fracture of the femoral shaft, hip, or lower leg; used with balanced-suspension traction

Thrombosis: Formation of thrombi inside a blood vessel or in a chamber of the heart

Thrombus: Blood clot formed in the heart or vessels from constituents of the blood

Traction: Application of a pulling force to an injured or disease body part

Transcondylar: Across or through the condyles

U

Ulceration: Formation of an ulcer on a body surface usually over a bony prominence

Bibliography

Bennett-Canclini S (1985). The kinetic treatment table: a new approach to bed rest, *Orthop Nurs* 4(2), 61–70.

Birmingham J (1992). *Discharge planning: a practitioner's guide to policies, procedures, and protocols.* Palos Verdes Estates Calif, Academy Medical Systems.

Browner CM, Hadley MN, Volker VKH, Mattingly LG (1987). Halo immobilization brace care: an innovative approach, *J Neurosci Nurs* 19(1), 24–29.

Carini GK, Birmingham JJ (1980). *Traction made manageable,* New York, McGraw-Hill.

Ceccio CM (1990). Understanding therapeutic beds, *Orthop Nurs* 9(3), 57–70.

Celeste S, Folcik MA, Dumas K (1984). Identifying a standard for pin site care using the quality assurance approach, *Orthop Nurs* 3(4), 17–24.

Cox HC, Hinz MD, Lubno, M.A., et al (1989). *Clinical applications of nursing diagnosis,* Baltimore, Williams & Wilkins.

Dunlop J (1939). Transcondylar fractures of the humerus in childhood, *J Bone Joint Surg* 21(1), 59–73.

Dunwoody CJ (1991). Pelvic fracture patient care, *Nurs Clin North Am* 26(1), 65–71.

Farrell J (1986). *Illustrated guide to orthopaedic nursing,* ed 3, Philadelphia, JB Lippincott.

Folcik MA, Ostnow MK (1990). Herniated nucleus pulposus. In *Patient teaching loose-leaf library,* Springhouse Pa, Springhouse Corp.

Hines NA, Bates MS (1987). Discharging the patient in skeletal traction, *Orthop Nurs* 6(4), 21–24.

Hirsch J, Anderson DR (1991). Pulmonary embolism. In Rakel RE (ed): *Conn's Current therapy,* Philadelphia, WB Saunders.

Howell E, Widra L, Hill MG (1988). *Comprehensive trauma nursing,* Glenview Ill, Scott Foresman.

Humphrey CJ (1986). *Homecare nursing handbook,* Norwalk Conn, Appleton-Century-Crofts.

Jones-Walton P (1988). Effects of pin care on pin reactions in adults with extremity fracture treated with skeletal traction and external fixation, *Orthop Nurs* 7(4), 29–33.

Karn MA, Ragiel CA (1986). The psychologic effects of immobilization on the pediatric orthopaedic patient, *Orthop Nurs* 5(6), 12–17.

Kerr A (1980). *Orthopaedic nursing procedures,* ed 3, New York, Springer Publishing.

Lowry TM (1934). The physics of Russell's traction, *J Bone Joint Surg* 17(1), 174–178.

Luchman J, Sorensen K (1987). *Medical-surgical nursing,* ed 3, Philadelphia, WB Saunders.

McCoullough FL (1989). Skeletal trauma in children, *Orthop Nurs* 8(2), 41–46.

Morris L, Kraft S, Tessem S, Reinisch S (1988). Special care for skeletal traction, *RN* (February), 24–29.

Mourad LA, Droste MH (1988). *The nursing process in the care of adults with orthopaedic conditions,* New York, John Wiley & Sons.

Newschwander GE, Dunst RM (1989). Limb lengthening with the Ilizarov external fixator, *Orthop Nurs* 8(3), 15–21.

Ohman K, Spaniol D (1990). Halo immobilization: discharge planning and patient education, *J Neurosci Nurs* 22(6), 351–357.

Olson B, Ustanko L (1990). Self-care needs of patients in the halo brace, *Orthop Nurs* 9(1), 27–33.

Osborne LJ, DiGiacomo I (1987). Traction: a review with nursing diagnoses and interventions, *Orthop Nurs* 6(4), 13–19.

Perry AG, Potter PA (1988). *Clinical nursing skills and techniques,* St Louis, Mosby.

Riley MAK, Beltran MJ (1986). *Clinical nursing inter-*

ventions with critical elements, New York, John Wiley & Sons.

Roaf R, Hodkinson LJ (1971). *Textbook of orthopaedic nursing,* Philadelphia, FA Davis.

Russell RH (1924). Fracture of the femur: a clinical study, *Br J Surg* 11, 491–502.

Salmond S, Mooney N, Verdisco L (eds) (1991). *National Association of Orthopaedic Nurses core curriculum for orthopaedic nursing,* ed 2, Pitman NJ, Anthony J Janetti.

Schoen DC (1986). *The nursing process in orthopaedics,* Norwalk Conn, Appleton-Century-Crofts.

Slye DA (1991). Orthopaedic complications, *Nurs Clin North Am* 26(1), 113–132.

Smith S, Duell D (1988). *Clinical nursing skills,* ed 2, Los Altos Calif, National Nursing Review.

Stearns CM, Brunner NA (1987). *Opcare. Orthopaedic patient care: a nursing guide,* vol 3, Pfizer Hospital Products Group.

Turek SL (1984). *Orthopaedics: principles and their applications.* ed 4, vol 2, Philadelphia, JB Lippincott.

Whaley LF, Wong DL (1989). *Essentials of pediatric nursing,* ed 3, St Louis, Mosby.

Zinola-Webb L, Berquist SL (1991). Standardized care plans for home care, *Home Healthcare Nurse* 8(6), 21–29.

Index

Skeletal traction, 9
  care of patient in, 43-45
  equipment for, 9-11
  to lower extremity and hip; *see* Lower extremity and hip, skeletal traction to
  maintaining proper position of patient in, 44
  positioning extremity in, 44
  to upper extremity; *see* Upper extremity, skeletal traction to
Skin, tenting of, at pin site, 47
Skin breakdown
  adjunct equipment to decrease risk of balanced-suspension traction and, 52
    Dunlop's traction and, 74
    external fixators and, 112
    general traction management and, 14
    overhead 90-90 traction and, 70
    sidearm traction and, 67
  increased risk of
    balanced-suspension traction and, 52
    general traction management and, 13-14
Skin care related to application of traction
  Dunlop's traction and, 75
  overhead 90-90 traction and, 71
  sidearm traction and, 68
Skin integrity
  alteration in
    Bryant's traction and, 30
    external fixator of pelvis and, 108
    external fixator on lower extremity and, 104-105
    patient in Kinetic Treatment Table and, 128
    pelvic sling and, 93-94
    pelvic traction and, 93-94
    skeletal cervical traction and, 87-88
    skeletal traction to lower extremity and hip and, 45-46
    skin and skeletal traction to upper extremity and, 61-62
    skin traction to lower extremity and hip and, 23-24
  Buck's traction and, 35
  impaired, potential for, in cervical traction, 79-80

Skin integrity—cont'd
  maintenance of
    balanced-suspension traction and, 52
    Boehler-Braun frame and, 131-132
    Bryant's traction and, 38
    cervical halter traction and, 97
    Dunlop's traction and, 73-74
    external fixators and, 112
    general traction management and, 13
    overhead 90-90 traction and, 70
    sidearm traction and, 66-67
    skeletal cervical traction and, 99
  and potential impairment caused by traction application to skin and prolonged bedrest, discharge planning and, 136
  Russell's traction and, 35
Skin traction, 8-9
  to lower extremity and hip; *see* Lower extremity and hip, skin traction to
  neurovascular dangers associated with, 29
  and skeletal traction to upper extremity; *see* Upper extremity, skin traction to
  to upper extremity, application of, 59-60
Sling
  Buck's traction and, 34
  pelvic; *see* Pelvic sling
  Russell's traction and, 34
Social services, traction in home setting and, 142
Spasms, traction and, 1-2, 3
Spine
  lumbar, circumferential skin traction to, 90, 91
  traction to, 76-101
    cervical traction, 76-83
    pelvic sling, 91-95
    pelvic traction, 90, 91
    skeletal cervical traction, 83-90
Splint
  Harris, 40
  Thomas; *see* Thomas splint
Spreader bar in pelvic sling, 101
Steinmann pin in skeletal traction, 9-10
Stockings, elastic, deep vein thrombosis and, 115

Straight leg raising exercises, 22
Straight-line traction, 40
Streptokinase, pulmonary embolism and, 118
Stryker frame, 85, 126-127
Supracondylar fractures of humerus in children, Dunlop's traction and, 58
Suspension, patient alignment and, in external fixators, 111

T

Tenting of skin at pin site, 47
Thomas splint, 40, 41-42
  leg in, with Pearson attachment in balanced-suspension traction, 51
  position of leg in, 42
Thrombolytic therapy, pulmonary embolism and, 118
Thrombophlebitis, 114-116
Thrombus, 114-116
Tibial nerve, assessment of, external fixator on lower extremity and, 105
Tissue perfusion, alteration in
  balanced-suspension traction and, 52
  Boehler-Braun frame and, 132
  Bryant's traction and, 38
  external fixators and, 112
  general traction management and, 14
Tongs, cervical, in skeletal traction, 10, 83, 98
Traction
  application of, 8-11
  balanced-suspension; *see* Balanced-suspension traction
  boots used in, 16, 20-21, 34, 115
  Bryant's; *see* Bryant's traction
  Buck's; *see* Buck's traction
  cervical; *see* Cervical traction
  cervical halter, care guide for, 96-97
  circumferential head halter, 76-83
  circumferential skin, to lumbar spine, 90, 91
  contractures and spasms and, 1-2
  definition of, 1-2
  discharge planning and; *see* Discharge planning
  divarication, 27-32
  Dunlop's; *see* Dunlop's traction